How to be Healthy with NATURAL FOODS

EDWARD E. MARSH

GRAMERCY PUBLISHING COMPANY • NEW YORK

To my children, Edward, Jane, Martha, Mary, Michael, and William, as well as to all those who read these words, my sincere hope that they may reap the benefits of life-long health and contentment.

FOREWORD

AS one progresses in natural growth and physical development, many times the idea of how to build up one's energy
and strength comes to mind. Although antibiotics and
widespread hygienic publicity have greatly diminished the
prevalence of infectious diseases and, on the whole, improved living conditions, appreciable numbers of Americans are still suffering from nutritional deficiencies. The
public gets little scientific information about wholesome
foods and less about the true source of health and well-
being. Thus very few people are mindful of the basic foods
needed to build a sound physical condition.

The collection of varied and specialized materials in
this book is startling. Many common fallacies about food
practices are exposed. This compact and comprehensive
presentation of practical information can revise any man's
notion of diet while correcting his theories of nutrition.
The author makes clear all the most important nutritional
data in a concise form, the fundamental principles of
which are put forth for consideration in a very interesting
style, chapter by chapter.

Truly, this book will alter your concept of food while
improving your ideas about health—teaching you how to
build up your energy and live.

JOHN P. URLOCK, JR., Ph.G., B.S., M.D.
President, Maryland Academy of
Medicine and Surgery

Baltimore, Maryland

PREFACE

Health is a crown on a well man's head, but no one can see it but a sick man.

—*Egyptian proverb*

IN recent decades man has made great progress in understanding and controlling the wonders of nature. In no field of human endeavor is his achievement more strikingly evident than in the sciences of nutrition and geriatrics.

In writing this book, it was my intention to set forth my thoughts, personal experience, and conclusions concerning modern nutritional knowledge and to show how the use of wholesome, natural foods can work to improve or restore mental and bodily health. There is nothing more important for human welfare than good health. I believe that illness is one of those events that should be opposed on principle.

Through actual trial and observation, I have long since discovered that one can maintain good health and eliminate colds and other minor ailments by the consistent use of specific foods and by excluding foods that are harmful in themselves or that contain nothing of nutritional value.

For this reason, I have put together in the pages that follow a summarized account of practical nutritional information, which sets forth in great variety the foods

5

that contain all the necessary proteins, carbohydrates, enzymes, fats, vitamins, and minerals. Readers can eliminate from their diet those items that they dislike or to which they may be allergic and still obtain the benefit of all the essential nutrients that build and maintain deepseated vitality, produce greater energy and strength, offer protection against premature senility, encourage more durable arteries, and promote health, well-being, and longevity. It is my ultimate purpose to present simple, tried and true principles, which have worked for me, for my family, and for many of my friends. THEY WILL WORK FOR YOU!

ACKNOWLEDGMENTS

I wish to pay tribute to all those who have given me inspiration, encouragement, and important assistance, as well as helpful criticism, during the preparation of this book.

I am particularly indebted to Mr. Philip M. Kellogg, Mr. Joseph Smith, and Mr. Samuel W. Nathanson, for their invaluable suggestions and advice. To them I owe much gratitude.

I also wish to thank, in a special way, Mrs. Nancy M. Gallienne, for scholarly editorial assistance, as well as the well-balanced treatment of the subject matter.

To Dr. John P. Urlock, who wrote the foreword, I offer my deep appreciation.

I am grateful to my daughter Martha for her kindness in typing the manuscript.

An expression of thanks is due the publishers who extended their permission to quote passages from books, magazines, and other source material.

Finally, I want to express cordial thanks to the librarians at the Enoch Pratt Library for their aid, so generously and so courteously given, and to the Special Diet Shop of Baltimore for all the help and advice extended to me there.

E. E. M.

CONTENTS

1

PAST AND PROLOGUE

IT is now generally recognized that it is not possible to attain a state of physical fitness or to stay free from disease and infirmity unless one eats the proper foods. However, little is achieved by mere recognition of this fact. Most people continue to take for granted that the human body is miraculously able to convert devitalized, highly processed foods into healthy tissue. Unfortunately, the average American is woefully ignorant of the fundamental principles of good nutrition and is unaware that faulty eating can do the body great harm.

Early in my search for better health, I became aware of the startling fact that many people chronically ill with degenerative diseases, such as arteriosclerosis, heart ailments, arthritis, diabetes, and nervous disorders, were young—in their late thirties, forties, and middle fifties. Upon reflection, I came to the conclusion that many of these people might have brought these ailments on themselves unwittingly through the kind of foods and beverages that they consumed. I resolved to find out if this were true and, if so, why—lest I myself become a victim.

When I began my research into the healing and health-giving properties of natural foods, my physical condition was such that I despaired of being able to continue to make provision for my family. For as long as I can recall, I had suffered from grave respiratory infections, which confined me at home for several weeks every year with dreadful chest colds. Three times during my life I was disabled with pneumonia, which further weakened my resistance to these attacks. On one of these occasions, I lost four months from work and, on another, an entire year. By the middle of 1958, my over-all health had begun to deteriorate, and I was feeling bone-weary most of the time. So, when I set out to study the nutritional approach to the problem, it was with the avowed purpose of doing something for myself in the way of physical renewal.

A prodigious amount of reading, combined with experimentation by trial and error, led me to the dramatic discovery that there is a miraculous healing power inherent in natural foods. After trying this, trying that, I was gradually able to work out a few basic, dependable rules for correct eating—and these rules worked! I learned that one can add to one's life expectancy by knowing which foods to use or to cut out of the dietary. These conclusions are supported by the findings of researchers in the field.

By adhering to these principles of nutrition, I regained my health and experienced a gradual increase in strength and vigor that exceeded my fondest expectations. I share these principles with you in this book, which is my testament of gratitude for renewed vitality, zest for living, and a full, happy life.

The human body is a marvelous, smoothly functioning instrument, which provides its own remedy for every disease that attacks it and which heals almost any impairment, if given a chance. For this reason, common sense suggests that the good Lord created human beings basically sound. Wishing us to be healthy and happy, He has bestowed upon all of us a much greater store of physical power than we ordinarily require. It is up to us to co-operate, so as to make the best use of this unique endowment. Even a moderate effort in this direction often makes the difference between success and failure—but you must make that effort!

Really good health is a state of genuine well-being, not simply the absence of disease. Unfortunately, however, many people have come to accept poor physical health as a normal part of life. In the course of my travels, handling accident and health insurance claims, which brings me into contact with many physicians, I encounter the practical application of this attitude wherever I go. All over the country—in large cities, small towns, and rural areas—doctors' offices and hospital clinics are flooded with patients. Although this would seem to be positive proof that the laws of health are being violated, many medical authorities would have us believe that there is not a thing to worry about. However, the flourishing business being done by physicians, hospitals, and convalescent homes unquestionably confirms the opinion of many influential nutritionists that the American people are the most over-wrought, overmedicated people in the world.

Expenditures for drugs and medicines in the United States are estimated to exceed four hundred million dollars a year. Even more is spent on blood builders, cold and influenza remedies, nasal sprays, and all kinds of pain killers and nerve tonics. Unfortunately, most of the money spent in this bewildered pursuit of health is money wasted. It is high time that people began to live in a manner so as to prevent sickness and ill health.

In a report on the health of the nation, Dr. W. Coda Martin, President of the American Academy of Nutrition, has stated:

There are many approaches to the prevention and treatment of such complex diseases, but there appears to be one common denominator as the basic cause of degenerative diseases. That one factor is malnutrition.[1]

Nutritional scientists and biochemists are demonstrating more clearly every day that most chronic diseases have their inception in defective eating habits, in excessive eating and drinking of harmful foods and beverages. This is confirmed in a recent report from the United States Department of Health, Education and Welfare, which states that 56 percent of Americans forty-five to fifty-five years of age suffer from chronic illnesses. The United States Public Health Service also announced (November 10, 1962) that, of the seventy-four million Americans who had a chronic disease of one kind or another, fifty-seven million were under sixty-five.

Degenerative conditions are no longer confined to older people. The over-all picture of health in the young man of draft age is rapidly deteriorating as revealed by the draft rejections from World War I to the Korean conflict, over a short period of thirty-two years. In World War I, 1918, 31.2 percent were not physically able for active military service. At this time the physical standards were high. In World War II, 1941 to 1943, the total found unfit for military service was about 41 percent. In the seven years from June, 1948, to June, 1955, some 52 percent of the young men called for preinduction examination were rejected for physical or mental defects—an increase of 11 percent over World War II, or a total of 21 percent increase in rejections since 1918 in spite of marked lowering of physical standards.[2]

[1] Testimony given to the Subcommittee on Health and Science of the House Committee on Interstate and Foreign Commerce by Dr. W. Coda Martin, President of the American Academy of Nutrition, on July 24, 1957.
[2] Robert Cummings, *Stay Young and Vital* (Englewood Cliffs, N.J.: Prentice-Hall, 1960).

A recent report on a ten-year survey of the eating habits of teenagers (who favor hot dogs, hamburgers, pizza pies, potato chips, and soft drinks) indicated that approximately three fourths of boys and girls between thirteen and nineteen are undernourished. No wonder, then that close to 20 percent of children under eighteen have some personality disorder or persistent physical defect, the most common being eye diseases, hearing complaints, and bad teeth. Most tragic of all—some four million of our young people are emotionally unsettled and confused.

An examination, for nutritional defects, of some fifty persons over age sixty, who were not confined to institutions, indicated that over 90 percent showed evidence of a deficiency of proteins and a shortage of vitamins A and C, as well as the essential minerals calcium and iron.[3] The well-known nutritionist, Adelle Davis, says that "people's diets are often partly inadequate in from twenty to sixty nutrients simultaneously."[4] Think about that for a moment.

To date, medical science has accomplished very little toward extending the life span of a sixty-year-old person. In 1900, for example, a man of sixty could anticipate an additional fourteen years. Today, despite all medical advances, a sixty-year-old man can look forward to another sixteen years of life: a trifling gain of only two years. In the United States, in spite of excellent medical facilities, first-rate housing, a strong economic system, and a progressive social security program, the ratios for physical and mental illness come close to being the highest in the world. Most of it can be traced to the meals consumed daily by almost every family in America.

But who is telling our people about health and how it

[3] Health and Nutrition News (December 1962).

[4] Adelle Davis, *Let's Eat Right to Keep Fit* (New York: Harcourt, Brace & World, 1954).

can be achieved? Why aren't we told by those who are supposed to know? Never, I believe, in the history of this nation have so much nonsense, so many half-truths and downright falsehoods been spread abroad about food.

The average American diet is high in refined carbohydrates, foods in which the B-complex vitamins are practically nonexistent. Processing of such foods also removes many important minerals, which provide vigor and help assure long life. It is reported that about 80 percent of the calories that we partake of every day, for the purpose of appeasing hunger, comes from inferior, processed foods.

To be healthy you must avoid the so-called "civilized foods," the refined and processed foods, such as white sugar, white bread and other bakery products, packaged cereals, ice cream, soft drinks, french fried potatoes, and the like. Eating such foods will assuredly bring about nutritional deficiencies and carries with it the added risk of their leading to serious disease.

The daily diet of most Americans is usually something like this. Breakfast consists of orange or grapefruit juice; a cold cereal with milk and sugar; toast with butter or margarine; and coffee, tea, or milk. Many people take only toast and coffee. For lunch, it's soup, generally canned, a hamburger or frankfurter on a roll or some other type of processed meat sandwich; coffee, tea, or milk, or a soft drink; and a dessert of cake, pie, or ice cream. Dinner usually comprises meat, potatoes, and cooked vegetables; a salad with dressing; bread with butter or margarine; canned fruit (often topped with whipped cream) or pie or ice cream; and coffee, tea, or milk.

The total daily food intake outlined above is grossly inadequate, leaving much to be desired in the way of substantial nourishment (especially breakfast). It is extremely low in energy-creating digestive enzymes. The good that may be obtained from the meats, vegetables, and fruits consumed is largely offset by the positive harm done the body by the bread, sugar, pastry, ice cream, and what have you, which are taken along with them. Consider now the between-meal snacks of potato chips, french fries, pretzels, pickles, crackers, and soft drinks, all loaded with salt, sugar, catsup, mustard, or relish. This unhappy situation is worsened by the addition of dangerous chemicals to the foods in the processing, a practice that has become so widespread in the industry that it is now almost impossible to obtain a commercial food product that has not been "doctored" in some way.

In the report cited previously, Dr. W. Coda Martin states, with respect to chemical additives:

> The human body can utilize only natural foods as nourishment and survive. Chemicals are not food elements. Therefore, they can produce only negative or harmful results, even though they are by scientific analysis non-toxic. It is then only a question of how much harm they will produce, when used to replace essential food elements in our diets.

There is every reason to believe that the American diet, with its inadequate benefits, has a definite effect upon the health of our people. The results can be seen everywhere— so many heavily burdened people, drifting wearily along the way to ill health, chronic disability, and premature death.

Contrast the all-too-typical daily food intake, outlined above, with the diet that follows. Since adopting this high-protein, high-fat, low-carbohydrate dietary, not only have I recovered my health, but I have more energy and endurance than I have enjoyed since I was a young man. In addition, the disabling diseases that had plagued me for years are a thing of the past. By maintaining the body's supply of protein and other necessary nutriments at an optimum level, I have been able to preserve my eyesight and hearing; my appetite and digestion are as wide awake as they were years ago; my blood pressure and pulse are within normal limits; and my physical and mental powers are unimpaired. Further, on my present fare, my weight does not vary by more than a pound or two from year to year.

UPON ARISING	One tablespoonful of apple cider vinegar and one tablespoonful of honey, dissolved in a glass of warm water
BREAKFAST	Stewed prunes Two eggs with bacon, ham, sausage, hamburger, or steak Black coffee
LUNCH	Cup of soup Hamburger steak or other meat Black coffee
DINNER	Tomato or vegetable juice (sometimes I have a glass of wine instead of juice) Choice of steak, liver, or other meat, or fish Baked or boiled potato A green or yellow vegetable or cottage cheese with fruit Black coffee
NIGHTCAP	Cup of yogurt with honey or fruit or sunflower seeds
SUPPLEMENTS	I supplement these foods with: Fifty thousand units of vitamin A and 3,400 units of vitamin D from fish-liver oil One tablespoonful each of brewer's yeast and of desiccated liver powder (for B-complex vitamins, additional protein, and minerals)

One or two tablespoonfuls of lecithin
granules (for unsaturated fatty acids)
Twelve hundred milligrams of vitamin C,
with the bioflavonoids, from rose hips
Six hundred units of vitamin E (D-alpha
tocopherol acetate only)
Eight Dolomite[5] and four bone-meal tablets (for magnesium and calcium)
Three kelp tablets (for iodine and trace
minerals)

Broadly speaking, you can promote good health by
following a simple plan, consisting of these four essentials:
follow a high-protein diet; get sufficient rest; keep the
inside of the body clean; and take frequent, moderate
exercise. Of the four, effective nutrition is unmistakably
the most important. There are no magical aids to a sound
physical condition. Health must be earned; it cannot be
had for the asking. Only by the regular, daily use of pure,
natural foods can it be attained.

In their younger years, most people enjoy buoyant
health and zest for living. Few, however, are able to maintain their abounding get-up-and-go after reaching the age
of fifty. This after-fifty setback may be due to improper
diet, provided no serious disease is present. Consequently,
if you are past fifty, you must begin to rebuild your body
if you wish to avoid senility and retain sound mentality
and physical vigor.

It is an amazing fact that it is within your power to
invigorate your mind and body and attain mental and
physical health at any age, as long as you supply the body
with the materials it needs to rebuild and repair the cells.
Specifically, you must follow a well-balanced diet, from
first to last, one that contains all the proper foods in the
amounts that are required for life and health. Bear in mind

[5] See p. 83.

that the human body can never be better than the food that it takes in daily to strengthen, revitalize, and rebuild it.

So the first big step is to re-examine your dietary habits, to make certain that you are obtaining enough of the indispensable elements of good nutrition. Cast off the food habits that are damaging and begin to use natural foods, which will give you powerful resistance to disease and guarantee a healthy body. You must start at once to eat plenty of meat, fish, eggs, and other high-protein foods and stop eating refined sugar, white flour, and their products. This is basic; it will make a big difference in the way you feel.

Read, then, the remarkable story of nutrition. If you have often been feeling listless and worn-out, the pages that follow will reveal unexpected ways to achieve well-being and zest for life. Let your fear and anxiety be replaced by knowledge and understanding. The plan proposed in this book is simple; it can be followed by anyone of any age. It involves neither drugs nor complicated regimens. And it promises rewards that are beyond price—the gifts of health, vitality, long life, and joy in living.

2

PROTEIN—BODY BUILDER

IN order for the human body to be healthy and strong and to have the stamina necessary for long life, it must have a liberal supply of basic foods and—just as important —it must be able to use them efficiently. Some foods are required for growth; others coordinate the ordinary bodily functions. One of the common causes of old-age symptoms is nutritional deficiency over a long period of time. Certain bodily functions become less vigorous as we grow older, and the aging person needs more of all nutriments than the younger one. This is particularly true with regard to protein. A man over fifty may require twice as much protein daily as does his grandchild.

Protein is the most vital of the food elements needed by the body. It is the foundation of protoplasm, the fundamental life-substance, from which all living organisms are formed. From the time you are born, every day of your life, you need protein to sustain life and growth, to form new tissues and cells, and to renew and rebuild those affected by the severity of daily living. The hemoglobin in your blood is 95 percent protein; your tissues, organs, skin, hair, and nails are mainly protein. Your bones and nerves are made of protein, as are the fluids secreted by the body—hormones and enzymes.

The body does not actually use proteins as such, but breaks them down into their components, which are called *amino acids*. These substances are found only in proteins; carbohydrates do not contain them. The digestive system separates the proteins in food into their component amino acids, which are then used by the body in many ways. Scientists have identified twenty-three different acids in food proteins. Only ten of these have been designated as indispensable, and must be secured from the food we consume; the body is able to develop the additional thirteen. Some nutritionists regard these essential amino acids as more important to health than vitamins and minerals, because it is obligatory to have them if you are to live out your normal term of years. They are a sort of blueprint for the structure of the cells.

Not every kind of protein will form good tissue. Animal proteins, such as meat, fish, eggs, and poultry, are known as complete proteins, since they include all ten of the essential amino acids in exact proportions for human nutrition. Vegetable proteins (with the exception of a very few foods, such as soybeans, sunflower seeds, and peanuts) do not contain all these essential acids in the correct amounts.

You will improve your health and lengthen your life in direct proportion to how faithfully you supply your body with complete protein, as well as with vitamins and minerals. When you know how to control the quality of your blood by a daily intake of the right kind of food and the right kind of liquid, you will possess a tremendous power over your health and life for good or ill.

When a protein deficiency exists, the liver becomes more liable to injury by toxic agents, resistance to infection is diminished, and wounds do not heal promptly. Edema, or waterlogging, is one of the commonest symptoms of a severe protein deficiency. Such a deficit is also one of the causes of anemia, high blood pressure, and retardation of growth. People who do not eat enough protein may not be actually sick, but they never feel truly well. The individual who complains of being tired all the time may very well be suffering from acute protein deficiency.

There is general agreement among leading nutritionists and food experts that a high-protein, high-fat, low-carbohydrate diet is essential for good health. The fact that virtually 60 percent of the protein consumed is changed into glucose in the body makes it unnecessary to use sugary foods, because a high-protein and high-fat diet will maintain normal blood-sugar levels.

Every day, make at least two thirds of your protein intake animal protein; the other third should be made up of fresh raw fruits, vegetables, nuts, and seeds. The emphasis should be on meat, fish, poultry, eggs, milk products, and soya products, since these are the only complete proteins. Seafood is also abundantly supplied with complete protein, in addition to the B vitamins and highly important minerals. This type of diet not only supplies the needed vitamins and minerals, but also moderates the tendency to head colds, pneumonia, and other respiratory ailments; helps disperse the intestinal gases caused by unabsorbed carbohydrate; and has a remarkable ability to protect the liver from damage.

The National Research Council has set an official recommendation that forty to one hundred grams of protein be eaten daily by growing children, depending upon their age. Seventy grams is suggested for mature persons. This is the lowest quantity necessary to provide protection against disease. The majority of nutritionists, however, urge a much higher daily intake. About twice the minimum, or one hundred forty grams, is usually recommended for superlative health and to bring about maximum resistance to illness.

The following table, listing the amount of protein in various foods, will help you estimate your daily consumption of this vital nutrient.

FOOD	QUANTITY	GRAMS OF PROTEIN
Bacon	3 slices	6
Brewer's yeast	1 heaping tablespoon	20
Cheese, American	1⅓ ounces	12
Cheese, cottage	½ cup	20
Chicken	4 ounces	18
Codfish	4 ounces	16
Eggs	1	6
Fish	4 ounces	21
Hamburger	4 ounces	19
Lamb chops	2	20
Lamb, roast	4 ounces	22
Lima beans	½ cup	8
Liver, beef or calf's	4 ounces	23
Milk, powdered	½ cup	35
Peas, dried	½ cup	12
Pork chops	4 ounces	23
Steak	4 ounces	30
Turkey	4 ounces	24

With these facts in mind, let us take a closer look at some of the most important protein foods available. The first of these is meat.

MEAT

The most significant thing about protein is quality, not quantity. This means protein containing all the principal amino acids in the right proportions. As stated previously, all the proteins containing the ten requisite amino acids are called first-class or complete proteins, and inasmuch as the organs of the body are practically entirely composed of protein, fresh meat is the most immediately available source of amino acids.

Another valuable food element in meat is its vitamin and mineral content (it is rich in iron). All meats, but especially the organ meats, are high in the B-complex vitamins.

In some places there is a prejudice against meat, but this originated in the days when an erroneous theory was proposed that meat and meat products caused dangerous toxic effects in the intestines. Properly cooked meats do not introduce harmful bacteria into the body, nor do they produce toxic effects in the digestive tract. As a matter of fact, animal protein has a much higher degree of digestibility than vegetable protein; so much so that meat is now a recommended food for babies.

In a healthy person, 97 percent of the protein in meat consumed is completely digested, while only 85 percent of the protein in cereal is digested, only 83 percent of vegetable protein, 78 percent of legume protein, and 85 percent of the protein in fruits.

Meat has been called "the wonderworking blood-builder and regenerator; assuager of epilepsy and migraine; the substance that favors rapid healing of wounds and of burns, that brings life to those dying of pernicious enemia, that protects the liver against injury from alcohol and disease, that helps overcome stammering, that cures pellagra, that aids recovery from tuberculosis, a nutritional necessity for the steady drinker and smoker."[1]

We should never forget that the ability to live well on a simple routine diet of meat and water is the common inheritance of mankind. It is only in the last five or six

[1] F. J. Schlink and M. C. Phillips, *Meat Three Times a Day* (Peterborough, N.H.: Richard R. Smith Co., 1946).

thousand years, since the Egyptians introduced cereals into the diet and man turned to agriculture, that trouble with tooth decay commenced.

It has been shown that decay in the teeth of the Eskimos was unknown before carbohydrates (sweets) were introduced to his diet.[2]

Arctic explorers have lived healthfully for as long as two years on meat, fat and lean, and nothing else. Vilhjalmur Stefansson, the famous arctic explorer, universally accepted as an authority on Eskimo life, with one of his companions, Karsten Andersen, spent a year (from February 1928 to March 1929) at Bellevue Hospital in New York, living on an exclusive diet of meat. At the end of the year, both men were physically active, mentally alert, and manifested no evidence of ill health.

Mr. Stefansson relates, in several of his books on life in the arctic, how almost all Eskimos are strict meat eaters, rarely eating any plant foods. As a result, arthritis, cancer, diabetes, tooth decay, and other degenerative diseases are virtually unknown among these people. They likewise have almost incredible powers of endurance. They eat heartily of walrus meat, including the fat, but are scarcely ever overweight.

LIVER

Meat has always been man's principal food and, as a rule, all meats contain the same amounts of the necessary amino acids. Brains, heart, kidneys, and liver, however, have a higher content of these vital acids.

It has long been known that liver of every type is an

[2] From a letter by Norman Highstein, D.D.S., to the Baltimore *Evening Sun,* April 1, 1963.

effectual source of complete protein, vitamin A, vitamin B-12 (it contains twenty to fifty times as much as muscle meats), and vitamin C—all indispensable to the body. It is also plentifully supplied with the minerals calcium, phosphorus, iron, copper, and iodine.

Of all natural protein foods, fresh liver is assuredly the most complete. Its substantial percentage of copper (which conserves iron), its full measure of all the amino acids, its reserve of all the other trace minerals, and the desirable B-complex elements unquestionably place liver as second to none of the build-up-your-energy foods.

Today, we know that liver is the most wholesome meat one can obtain. Desiccated liver, which is a concentration of whole liver in powder form, is a close second to fresh liver. Two heaping tablespoons are equivalent to one serving, or one quarter pound of meat, and supplies 12½ grams of high-quality protein.

Its numerous functions are amazing. For example, even small amounts of liver help the body eliminate DDT and strychnine and will neutralize the effects of cortisone, the sulfa drugs, and many other dangerous chemical substances. It has a powerful effect in regulating at least some of the functions of the reproductive system. It also helps relieve fatigue.

Using desiccated liver is a simple, easy way to get an unfailing supply of the vitamins, minerals, amino acids, and other constituents so abundant in fresh, uncooked liver. It is also available in tablet form. It is advisable to have liver at least once or twice a week.

FATS

No one can live without fats. Why? First, fats contain fatty acids and vitamins essential for health. Second, fats are a centralized source of heat and energy, which the body requires for its mode of operation. Third, fats provide reinforcement, because they slow down the rate at which food is digested. Fourth, fats, when stored in the body in reasonable amounts, produce an energy reserve, a cushion for vital organs, and insulation against excessive temperatures. And last, but not least, they improve the flavor of a meal.

Possibly by this time you are wondering about the relationship between meat and meat fat and the much-talked-about cholesterol. Be assured, however, that meat fats have little effect on the cholesterol level. Even if meat fat did step up cholesterol, it is not generally recognized that cholesterol is an integral part of all living cells. Cholesterol is also closely related to vitamin D, which prevents rickets and is part of the bile acids and sex hormones.

FISH

Man has eaten fish and other products of the sea since prehistoric times. Fish is practically a perfect food, and all over the world it constitutes a major part of man's diet. It is an excellent source of high-quality protein, vitamins, and minerals. It is low in fats, and the fats present are furnished liberally with polyunsaturates. Where fish and other seafood are a substantial part of the dietary, goiter and anemia are virtually unheard of.

Many foods today are robbed of their vitamins and minerals by processing, and, in addition, contain residues of insecticides. Fishes and other marine life feed on primitive substances, developed and sheltered by nature so that man cannot interfere.

The expectant mother can benefit her unborn child through the plentiful quota of calcium, copper, fluorides, iodine, iron, magnesium, and phosphorus contained in all seafoods. Anyone desiring to preserve their arteries in a good state of health can do so by eating fish and other marine foods frequently.

Popular kinds of fish and other seafoods are clams, crabs, fresh mackerei, flounder, haddock, halibut, lobster, oysters, scallops, shrimp, sole, trout, and tuna. The meat is tender and up to 95 percent digestible.

EGGS

Eggs are another superior protein food that is known to be of the highest biological benefit, the most perfect protein in the human diet. They contain all the amino acids in generous amounts—even more liberally than meat. One or two eggs a day are recommended for everyone.

Eggs also offer more and finer valuable nutrients for producing and sustaining body tissues than any other food —more vitamin A, thiamine (B-1), D, E, and niacin than most foods. Further, they supply a full measure of minerals, such as calcium, magnesium, and phosphorus.

It is true that eggs do contain cholesterol, but they are also an excellent source of lecithin, inositol, choline, methionine, threonine, and other effective cholesterol-controlling agents, which assist in keeping cholesterol in solution in the bloodstream.

POWDERED MILK

Powdered milk is an elementary food, an exceptional source of protein, calcium, riboflavin (this B vitamin is one of the principal factors in delaying the aging process), and many other nutrients. It is one of the most concentrated, economical, tasteful, and best assimilated of all protein foods.

The outstanding merit of powdered milk consists in its abundance of fat-free protein, vitamins B-1 (thiamine), B-2 (riboflavin), B-6 (pyridoxine), B-12, choline, inositol, niacin, pantothenic acid, para-amino-benzoic acid, biotin, and folic acid, plus all the minerals necessary for human health. An analysis of powdered milk indicates that it contains a high concentration of the minerals calcium, chlorine, cobalt, copper, iodine, iron, magnesium, manganese, phosphorus, potassium, sodium, sulphur, and zinc: more than most other foods.

Since a great many older people are not up to normal levels in protein, calcium, riboflavin (B-2), and other vitamins of the B-complex, powdered milk serves as an ideal rejuvenator for the heart, brain, and nerves, and generally to strengthen the failing body.

An inexpensive, effective way of getting increased quality protein in the diet is to add a couple of tablespoonfuls of powdered milk to custards, sauces, soups, scrambled eggs, hamburgers, and similar foods. Only one-half cup will deliver thirty-five grams of high-grade protein to the diet, which is equivalent to the protein in six eggs.

A BASIC DIET

It is better for your health to keep your meals simple. Meat, fish, or eggs; one or, at the most, two side vegetables; and a beverage, is suitable fare for most people. If you want a dessert, eat fresh fruit or cottage cheese, or, better still, combine the two. By adding appropriate vitamin and mineral supplements, you can assure yourself of proper nourishment.

Beans, cheese, eggs, fish, fresh vegetables, fruits, lentils, meats, nuts, poultry, seeds, and whole grains are the foods that build stamina and endurance. When too much sugar and starch is consumed, instead of these protective foods, malnutrition and nervous collapse are not far off. Wholesome food preserves health and also prevents or aids in the cure of disease. Unless you follow a sound basic diet, vitamin and mineral supplements cannot do all the work.

The more I study and observe, the more convinced I become that planned nutrition can prevent premature aging. People grow older very rapidly on refined and nonvital low-protein diets. If one will apply the known facts, the specter of old age may be held off for many years.

No doubt you have heard all your life the admonition to chew your food well. What may surprise you is the fact that protein foods such as those mentioned above need little chewing for good digestion. Organized observation conducted to put this theory to the test has indicated that protein foods that are swallowed in sizable, compact portions will be digested very much better than will the same foods that have been overcooked, ground up, or masticated thoroughly. The stomach acids do the actual work of digesting these proteins.

On p. 32 you will find lists of animal and vegetable protein foods, as well as low-carbohydrate fruits, which you can use as a guide to plan your daily diet.

Animal proteins:

beef	honey	salmon
brains	kidney	sardines
cheese	lamb	scallops
chicken	liver	shad
cottage cheese	lobster	shad roe
crabmeat	milk, whole	shrimp
eggs	oysters	steak
fish	pork	tunafish
heart	yogurt	turkey

Limited list of vegetable proteins:

almonds	cucumbers	parsley
asparagus	dates	parsnips
beets	eggplant	peanuts
brewer's yeast	figs	peas
broccoli	green peppers	potatoes, white
brown rice	kale	sesame seeds
brussels sprouts	lentils	squash
cabbage	lettuce	string beans
carrots	lima beans	sunflower seeds
cauliflower	navy beans	tomatoes
celery	olives	turnips
corn	onions	wheat germ

Low-carbohydrate fruits:

apples	currants	peaches
apricots	gooseberries	pears
avocado	grapes	pineapple
blackberries	honeydew melon	plums
blueberries	huckleberries	prunes
cantaloupe	lemons	raspberries
cherries	limes	strawberries
cranberries	loganberries	watermelon

ENZYMES

The chemical agents called enzymes are minute catalysts, all made of protein and containing all the essential amino acids. Those intricate chemical elements, which are produced within our bodies, are indispensable factors for life itself and are necessary for carrying on the work of the cells.

Enzymes accomplish astonishing tasks of biological composition and perform an infinite number of life-sustaining chain reactions with remarkable efficiency. In other words, they break down food as it passes through the alimentary canal and are responsible for its digestion, thereby aiding in the changing of food into blood, tissue, and energy.

Enzymes are only available in raw, uncooked foods, as their potency is cancelled out by heat. Be sure to include in your diet some or all of the following foods:

apple cider vinegar	milk, unpasteurized
brewer's yeast	nuts
cabbage	onions
fruits, raw	pineapple
garlic	royal jelly
honey	vegetable oils (unrefined)
liver, desiccated	vegetables, green leafy
meat (medium cooked)	yogurt

In concluding this section on quality proteins, I would suggest that the beginning of nutritional wisdom is to keep your menu plain and nutritious. In this way, you will obtain a balanced food assortment, containing substantial amounts of proteins, vitamins, minerals, and enzymes, while permitting the digestive processes to operate harmoniously. This is the type of diet that has proved successful in my own case—and in that of many persons I know—in improving or restoring health.

3

WHOLESOME CARBOHYDRATES

WHEN I began my own search for better health and physical reconditioning, I very soon became suspicious of the effects of adulterated, refined, and processed foods. By that I mean factory-created and mass-produced edibles such as bread and bakery products of all kinds, white sugar and substances made with it, ice cream, packaged cereals and mixes, soft drinks, french fried potatoes, potato chips, and so forth. Many chemicals are added to these foods without their having been tested beforehand to verify their safety. These food items are generally those from which you should be especially careful to abstain. Remember that using sugary and starchy foods to excess tends to lower the blood-sugar level, which produces heart and circulatory symptoms.

Of course, not all carbohydrates should be avoided. Some of them are valuable to health, because they contain natural vitamins, minerals, and enzymes. Natural carbohydrates, in combination with fats, sustain and invigorate the body and supply warmth and vitality. They cannot, however, take the place of protein, so make certain to obtain carbohydrates in foods that also contain a high degree of protein, vitamins, and minerals.

POTATOES

The potato is one of the three great foods whose natural home is the Western Hemisphere. The tomato and corn are the other two.

Potatoes are not included in the group of starches to be excluded from a high-protein meal, because this vegetable contains such primary nutritional elements as vitamins B-1 (thiamine), B-2 (riboflavin), niacin, vitamin C, and the mineral iron. It appears that carbohydrate cannot be utilized profitably unless it is in combination with the B vitamins, and potatoes are therefore one of the best sources of carbohydrates.

Potatoes, in common with almost all vegetables, supply a higher proportion of alkaline mineral elements than any other class of foodstuff, and therefore their consumption helps to maintain an alkaline reserve in the body. The raw potato is the most alkaline or anti-acid of all vegetables, due to the very high proportion of potassium. Further, potatoes contain the all-important vitamin C, which places them among what nutritionists call the protective foods. . . .

The potato is very easily digested because the starch of which it is largely composed is very loosely combined with the cellulose, or vegetable fibre, which constitutes the framework, or substance, of the tubers. Because of this digestibility, the potato is readily assimilated. It can be eaten freely without detriment.[1]

---

[1] Dr. H. Valentine Knaggs, *Potatoes as Food and Medicine* (Ashingdon, Rochford, Essex, England: The C. W. Daniel Co., 1958).

HONEY

The first one of the superior sugars that comes to mind is honey. It is one of the most perfect foods known. Honey is a vitamin-, mineral-, and enzyme-bearer, as well as a fine natural sweetener. Since the heart works on sugar, honey is the best heart stimulant you can use. It is in the bloodstream in twenty minutes after being taken by mouth, and this rapid absorption prevents fermentation. Because of its high sugar content, it will not spoil, even if exposed to contamination.

It is interesting to note that, while most body cells can receive some food from other sources, the nutriment of the brain is exclusively glucose. Blood sugar, then, is as critical to life as the air we breathe. It is the fuel of the body. Carbohydrates, such as honey, are highly important in the diet if the blood-sugar level is to be kept up to normal. This is where honey has the advantage over sugars having greater amounts of dextrose, because it does not cause the blood-sugar level to climb higher than can be handled by the body.

There does not appear to be any doubt that the first use of honey dates back beyond human records. It is probable that honey-bees and their products precede the appearance of mankind in time. The long chronicle of written history reveals that, for the past six thousand years, honey has been the only sweetener used by man, as well as his favorite sweetmeat and tonic. Honey is often mentioned in the Bible as a beneficial medicine, a health-giving food, and an element of delicious refreshment. It fills any void that may occur in the daily food intake.

Hippocrates, a Greek physician, known as the "Father of Medicine," was born about four hundred fifty years before Christ. In his medical practice he placed great reliance on diet and therapy, and many of his teachings are adhered to at the present day. He was a believer in honey and used it himself. He advocated it for those who wished to live long and for troublesome breathing.

In former ages honey had a notable reputation for imparting clearer eyesight. People in ancient times had firm faith in the potency of honey to increase stamina and manly vigor. From the Middle Ages down to our own times, honey has been more in favor, especially in rural areas, as a curative substance than the learned profession of medicine might suspect.

Honey has three fine qualities: it is a wholesome food; it is a purifying cleanser; and it has regenerative power.

In cases of pneumonia and typhoid fever, where digestive functions are below par, honey is of considerable value. It is a favored remedy for hay fever, nasal sinusitis, and throat and bronchial complaints. It is a fine expectorant and soothes irritation. It also benefits intestinal ulcers and gall bladder disease. It is said that there is no cancer or paralysis among bee-keepers.

The medicinal qualities of honey are impressive: for example, when disease bacteria come into contact with honey, vital moisture is withdrawn from them by the potassium in the honey, and they are destroyed. The acid reaction of honey also makes it a poor medium for the breeding of disease bacteria. Hostile germs that attack the body are, for the most part, exterminated in honey.

Honey is predominately fruit sugar, and is the only animal carbohydrate suitable for use as a sweet. It is one of the few sweets that has natural laxative qualities.

Also included in honey are enzymes, so necessary for

good digestion, and for this reason it is valuable for persons afflicted with anemia or chronic indigestion, convalescents, or the aged.

It is a tissue- and an energy-builder, chock-full of the material the body requires to construct and rebuild itself, an admirable restorative for all-round physical improvement.

According to the United States Department of Agriculture, honey is a general dietary source of the following nutrients:

> levulose (fruit sugar)
> dextrose (grape sugar)
> sucrose (cane sugar)
> water
> dextrins and gums

B-complex vitamins

B-1 (thiamine)   folic acid
B-2 (riboflavin)   niacin
biotin   pantothenic acid

> B-6 (pyridoxine)
> vitamin C
> vitamin K

Minerals

aluminum   manganese
calcium   phosphorus
chlorine   potassium
copper   silicon
iron   sodium
magnesium   sulphur

LACTOSE

Another valuable sugar is lactose, which is found only in milk. Lactose provides food for the beneficial intestinal bacteria, which convert it into lactic acid. This substance does not ferment, as do the carbohydrates in foods such as spaghetti, rice, white flour, refined sugar, and alcohol. It is one of the rare carbohydrates that actually promote the body's ability to absorb vitamins B-2 and B-6, and the minerals calcium and phosphorus. It leads to the multiplication of the beneficial bacteria in the large intestine, thus fostering a clean, healthy condition, which helps overcome the disease variety of bacteria that cause gas fermentation and sickness.

CAROB POWDER

Another excellent product, which can be used as a sweetener and also as a substitute for chocolate, is carob powder. It is a properly balanced, natural source of calcium, iron, magnesium, phosphorus, potassium, and other important minerals and vitamins.

According to the United States Department of Agriculture:

> Carob or St. John's Bread (*Ceratonia siliqua*) is a handsome evergreen tree which belongs to the . . . bean family. Known to man since antiquity, it has been cultivated in the Mediterranean region throughout historical times. It is the "St. John's Bread" of Christian tradition, a name derived from the fact that it was supposedly the food of John the Baptist during his sojourn in the wilderness. . . . The seeds are said to be the original carat weight of goldsmiths.

Carob powder is obtainable in health food and diet shops.

4

VITAMINS—NATURE'S SPARK PLUGS

THE "vital spark of life" is that awesome and stupendous faculty that all living things possess. Animals and plants have this power, the power to grow and reproduce their kind. Your body, too, is endowed with this living force, but it must be supported and preserved by the intake of foods that contain all the nourishment that the body requires.

Vitamins are an integral part of an enzyme that aids digestion, and they act as catalysts, which help to control metabolic processes. In other words, they help in the assimilation of the food you eat by contributing the element that changes fats, starches, and sugars into energy. Vitamins convert protein into amino acids for tissue repair and development. They help the mucous membranes to resist disease germs; they give strength to blood vessels and capillaries and feed nerve cells. Without enough of them, metabolic processes cannot progress in a normal manner, and poor health and exhaustion result.

Are all vitamins the same? By no means. They are either natural or synthetic. Natural organic vitamins supply all the related nutritional factors; and each of the various vitamins, in its own way, promotes health and keeps one feeling hale and hearty. The synthetic vitamins are segregated chemical elements usually made from coal-tar derivatives.

Vitamins in their natural state are found in food, in accurate proportions, functioning together interdependently, and also associated with many other substances as yet unidentified. But, due to processing, adulterating, handling, and shelf storage, many foods obtained in modern markets are sorely deficient in the vitamins that the body must have for development and proper functioning. Because of the widespread overrefinement of foods (which destroys these vital substances) you must take vitamin supplements to restore the missing components.

For this reason, a generous supply of all the basic vitamins should be furnished intensively and persistently, because omission of these elements leads to physical failure. This is especially true with older persons.

As for how much, this is a matter that only you can decide after evaluating the facts of nutrition you have learned. What is adequate or even bountiful for one person may be grievously meager for another. My experience has taught me that one has to experiment a bit to determine the individual potencies that are needed. You must learn to analyze your own condition.

Therefore, pay heed to your daily menu and make sure that it provides all known nutrients in full measure—all fats, minerals, natural sugars, vitamins, and proteins. Remember—food supplements give a lift, so to speak, but natural, wholesome food itself is more essential.

VITAMIN A

Vitamin A is a fat-soluble vitamin (that is, it dissolves in fat), and it can be stored in the body. This vitamin is extremely valuable for the health of the linings of the ears, lungs, mouth, nose, throat, and all body organs, and is indispensable for healthy bones and tooth enamel, good appetite, and normal digestion, reproduction, and lactation (the formation and secretion of breast milk).

Vitamin A is essential for healthy skin and bright, clear eyes. It protects against deterioration of the skin, as well as contributing to the well-being of the salivary glands, the ovaries, and the prostate. If one follows good nutrition, infections of the prostate gland can be avoided. If a prostate infection does occur, the diet should be enriched with supplements of vitamins A and C and vegetable oils. Research has also shown that vitamin A is of particular value as a deterrent of infections, such as habitual colds. Substantial amounts of the vitamin have been found in the relief of hay fever. It has also been found to be helpful in treating ear complaints, firming loose teeth, relieving aching corns and calluses on the feet, and improving the condition of people with goiter or other thyroid ailments.

Few people are aware that this vitamin lowers the cholesterol level in the blood. "Still fewer know that in a report in the *Medical Journal of Australia,* August 19, 1961, vitamin A was found to reduce by 60 percent the incidence of coronary heart disease, and to reduce by 90 percent the severity of coronary attacks."[1]

The earliest symptoms of vitamin A deficiency are usually noticed as night blindness and sensitivity to bright light. The first changes in the skin are dryness and roughness; the hair lacks sheen and luster; dandruff accumulates; fingernails easily break and peel. A deficiency of this food substance is also one of the causes of stones in the bladder and kidneys, as well as in the pulp of the teeth. It can likewise cause a loss of the sense of taste.

---

[1] *Health and Nutrition News* (December 1962).

The recommended minimum daily requirement of vitamin A is four thousand international units. From studies made by Dr. Henry C. Sherman, of Columbia University, it appears that an intake of four or five times this amount could increase the life span by 15 or 20 percent. The survey disclosed that persons with greater quantities of vitamin A in the blood have a lower mortality rate than those with lesser amounts of this substance.

Probably the most satisfactory and least expensive source of vitamin A is liver. Fish liver oils, too, are especially well supplied with vitamin A and D, in the proportional relation in which they are needed.

Other good sources are:

apricots	dandelion greens	prunes
asparagus	egg yolk	soybeans
broccoli	kale	spinach
butter	kidneys	squash, yellow
cantaloupe	lettuce	string beans
carrots	milk, whole	sunflower seeds
celery	mustard greens	sweet potatoes
chard	parsley	tomatoes
cheese	peaches	turnip greens
collards	peas	watercress
corn, yellow	persimmons	

VITAMIN B-COMPLEX

The importance of obtaining all the B-complex elements in your diet cannot be exaggerated. They fortify your nerves against the burdens and pressures of daily living. They are required for high energy. They are water-soluble vitamins, and must be replaced every day, as the body cannot store them.

We are intended to get our vitamins from the food we

eat, and so food comes first, because it is the primary source of all nourishment. Let us realize, then, with respect to the B vitamins at least, that our body demands must be met by nutritious foods. If you do not do this consistently, vitamin and mineral supplements will not be of much value.

There are some fifteen members of the B-complex family that have been identified. In view of the fact that they are poorly provided for in the American dietary, almost everyone needs them. Almost two thirds of the calories we eat are distributed among foods that have had a goodly portion of their natural nutrients eliminated. Eating white sugar, drinking excessively, and smoking also swindle you of B vitamins. Baking powder and baking soda neutralize these vitamins. If you are puzzled as to why you always feel tired, ponder the possibility that your vitamin B supply is too low.

The B vitamins are definitely effective in correcting defective digestion and improving the skin, mouth, tongue, arteries, nerves, eyes, and liver. They are absolutely essential to the heart's vigorous power, and are also vital for well-regulated elimination. This group of vitamins improves health in numerous ways. They are a must for a healthy body.

If you want to increase the body's ability to cope with stress, stop damaging accumulations of cholesterol from forming in the arteries, protect yourself against cancer, and produce immunity to many diseases, include plenty of the B-complex vitamins in your diet. All of them are of the utmost importance, because without these vitamins in at least the minimum amounts, life cannot be supported.

Another function of the B-complex vitamins is to assist in developing the digestive acids of the stomach. One of the essential requirements for a long and healthy life is a strongly acid stomach. As we grow older, we tend to have less hydrochloric acid in the stomach than younger people. Hydrochloric acid secretion is normal when the B vitamins, especially vitamin B-1 (thiamine) and niacin, are procured in sufficient quantity. These vitamins are the best guarantee of adequate hydrochloric acid in the stomach, which in turn prevents disease-threatening bacteria from getting into the intestines.

Stomach acidity can be sustained by taking apple cider vinegar or eating garlic or onions. Dry table wines, such as burgundy, claret, Rhine wines, and sauterne also aid digestion in this way. Such wines contain 10 to 12 percent alcohol, which is more than is present in beer and ale, but they also contain less carbohydrate.

No two individuals have identical requirements of these vitamins. Body structure, whether it be large or small, and physical activity determine one's needs, and these demands can be considerably affected by excessive perspiration in summer as well as by stress.

A deficiency in the B vitamins breeds malnutrition, enlargement of the heart, atrophy of muscles, loss of appetite, and failure to grow. Further, it may lead to personality defects, such as loss of self-confidence and lowered morale, which in turn can produce nervous tension.

Some symptoms of a vitamin B deficiency are:

beriberi	insomnia
burning and dryness of the eyes	lack of appetite
burning sensation in the feet	nausea
colitis	neuritis
constipation	nervousness
cracks at the corners of the mouth	pellagra
depression	serious defects in memory
diarrhea	shortness of breath
fatigue	skin disorders
fatty liver	sore tongue
headache	tender gums
indigestion	

The two most fruitful sources of the whole B-complex are brewer's yeast and liver. Other foods in which B vitamins are plentiful are:

berries	heart	soybeans
cheese	kidneys	sunflower seeds
egg yolk	legumes	wheat germ
fish	melons	whey
fowl	milk, whole	whole grains
fruits	peanuts	yogurt

All component parts of the B-complex are mutually dependent and are so vital to health and well-being that they all should be taken at the same time, since taking only one or more single vitamins can cause a deficiency in the others. Be wary, therefore, of the risky, lopsided, B-complex formulas so universally accepted today.

THIAMINE (VITAMIN B-1)

Thiamine, or vitamin B-1, is precisely related to the activity of the nervous system and is the chief nerve relaxant of all the B vitamins. A lingering scarcity of this vitamin may indeed cause a breakdown of the myelin sheath, which covers the nerve endings.

Vitamin B-1 is the food factor that improves your proficiency to absorb knowledge, promotes a calm nervous system (which, in one sense, is the very basis of health), gives you a feeling of confidence and self-respect, and enables you to meet difficulties with assurance.

This vitamin is required by the body to burn glucose and helps to convey vital oxygen to where it is needed. The older you are, the more thiamine you need. You also require vitamin B-1 for normal appetite and orderly digestion.

An insufficiency of vitamin B-1 causes fatigue, gas, heart trouble, insomnia, low thyroid activity, neuritis (which sometimes assumes the characteristics of lumbago, neuralgia, sciatica, or shingles), shortness of breath, and severe weakness. Even slight deficiencies can affect your normal temperament adversely, causing such personality changes as depression, inability to stand noise, jealousy, lack of interest, loss of morale, and nervous tension.

Potent sources of this vitamin are:

beef	heart	peas
blackstrap molasses	kidney	pork
brains	legumes	rice polishings
brewer's yeast	lentils	sardines
chicken	liver	soybeans
codfish	milk, powdered	sunflower seeds
dry beans	mutton	wheat germ
eggs	nuts	whole grains
fish roe	peanuts	yogurt

RIBOFLAVIN (VITAMIN B-2)

This important member of the B-complex is necessary for general health and energy, and is particularly necessary in order to help the cells in the tissues exchange oxygen, to keep vision undimmed, and to maintain clear skin and healthy hair. It is said that this vitamin is specifically required to foster superior resistance to disease, produce sturdy descendants, and increase longevity.

Riboflavin, or vitamin B-2, in combination with vitamin A, inhibits night blindness, which threatens airplane pilots and drivers of automobiles. Abnormal sensitivity to bright light, irritation and fatigue of the eyes, and soreness of the mouth, nostrils, and ears may be corrected when treated with this substance.

One of the first symptoms of vitamin B-2 deficiency appears as alterations of the visual apparatus of the eye, causing clouded vision. The whites of the eyes become bloodshot; sometimes there is granular inflammation; and the eyes water readily. As lack of riboflavin is considered to be the greatest single vitamin deficiency in our country today, make it a point to get a substantial amount of this element every day.

A greater intake of vitamin B-2, through the use of brewer's yeast, liver, and yogurt, will usually clear up any visual symptoms or other signs of deficiency. Eggs, green leafy vegetables, rice polishings, and wheat germ are other foods in which vitamin B-2 is present in good quantity.

PYRIDOXINE (VITAMIN B-6)

Pyridoxine, or vitamin B-6, is another very important element of the B-complex that, among other services, aids in conserving protein and in keeping your nerves young. A remarkable natural tranquilizer, it is winning distinction for its calming and comforting effect on the nervous system.

Extraordinary effects have been achieved by supplying vitamin B-6 to persons afflicted with epilepsy, hand tremors, insomnia, nervousness, palsy, or St. Vitus's dance. I wish to note here, however, that epilepsy, as such, cannot be cured by vitamin B-6, but seizures can be warded off or alleviated. It is a powerful food, rather than a drug.

Pyridoxine (vitamin B-6) is a muscle strengthener; consequently, it has proven useful in treating assorted types of muscular rigidity and distressing stiffness of the legs. It is likewise important to the utilization of fats, the forming of blood, the harmonious operation of muscles, and the health of the skin; and it has some bearing on the growth, color, and texture of the hair. It also improves human tolerance to noise.

Reports indicate that the greasy type of dandruff, as well as oiliness of the skin, so prevalent among acne sufferers, are greatly benefited, and occasionally vanish entirely, after a short period of treatment with vitamin B-6. It seems obvious that the oil glands of the skin cannot work properly without this substance. This may be a clue to why B-6 has been found effective in protecting sun-sensitive persons.

Some of the consequences of an insufficiency of vitamin B-6 in the diet are air- and sea-sickness, dizziness, lessened resistance to middle-ear infection, inferior muscle strength, and skin disease.

Since vitamin B-6 is purged from grains in the refining process, it may be found liberally supplied in the following foods:

beets	fish	muscle meats
blackstrap molasses	heart	nuts
brains	honey	peanut oil
brewer's yeast	kidney	rice polishings
cabbage	legumes	seeds
corn oil	liver	wheat germ
egg yolk	milk, whole	whole grains

VITAMIN B-12

Vitamin B-12 was at first called "the animal protein factor," because it is only available in animal sources.

Vitamin B-12 restrains and checks degeneration of cells in the central nervous system and, with the help of iron, aids in the prevention of cell deterioration. It affords a successful treatment for a sore tongue, aids bronchial asthma and extreme fatigue, helps treat varying degrees of deafness, and has relieved migraine headaches when everything else has proved disappointing. Massive doses have been used to ease the pain of neuritis.

It is said that vitamin B-12 encourages growth in underdeveloped children who have shown no improvement with other treatments. But where this vitamin has demonstrated its greatest power is in the treatment of the deadly pernicious anemia.

A want of B-12 also causes difficulties in muscular coordination and harmful mutations in the bone marrow.

Liver is the best source of this vitamin, but it can also be obtained in brewer's yeast, kidneys, milk, and wheat germ.

BIOTIN

Biotin, every so often referred to as the "mental health vitamin," is an extraordinarily effective stimulant to the development of healthy cells, and is, therefore, vital to sound nourishment of the body, as well as being important to general growth. It is also required so that fat can be digested and assimilated.

Biotin deficiencies result in unusual fatigue, dry, peeling skin, mental distress, muscular pain, uneasiness in the heart region, poor appetite, and upset stomach.

Good sources are:

brewer's yeast	liver
egg yolk	tomatoes
kidneys	wheat germ

CHOLINE

Choline is one of the B vitamins that controls the distribution of food fats throughout the body and aids gall bladder functioning. As choline is serviceable in helping to retard hardening of the arteries and diseases related thereto, it lessens the possibility of heart attacks.

This substance is also needed by the kidneys, for lactation in nursing mothers, and for the spleen; and it has been employed successfully in medical care of cirrhosis of the liver. It is also used for treating diabetes, glaucoma, and muscular dystrophy.

Valuable food sources are:

brains	lecithin granules	snap beans
brewer's yeast	liver	soybeans
cabbage	meat	spinach
egg yolk	mustard greens	tongue
fish	peas	turnip greens
fruits	rice polishings	wheat germ
heart	root vegetables	whole grains
kidney		

FOLIC ACID

Folic acid has been found necessary in moderate quantities in order for the bone marrow to make red blood cells of average size and normal number. It aids in the treatment of certain varieties of anemia, in particular the dread pernicious anemia. Folic acid is necessary for normal liver activity and has some bearing on preserving natural hair coloring.

A lack of this vitamin brings about proneness to intestinal parasites and food poisoning. Insufficiency also causes fatigue, pallor, weakness, and, ultimately, anemia.

Folic acid is abundant in:

brewer's yeast	liver
eggs	meat
fowl	mushrooms
fruits	oysters
grains, sprouted	soybeans
green leaves, uncooked	wheat germ
kidneys	

INOSITOL

Inositol is one of the B vitamins that is basic to life, but of which all the benefits to the body are not yet known. It is, however, most valuable for normal intestinal activity, especially the metabolism of fats; health of the skin; and hair growth and color. It is found in very small amounts in all the cells of the body. It is especially localized in the heart muscle and the lens of the eye.

Inositol is used to advantage in treating cerebral palsy, diabetes, gall bladder disease, multiple sclerosis, muscular dystrophy, and other ailments of the muscles and nerves. This vitamin also combines with choline to maintain cholesterol in suspension, and it helps the body to make use of vitamin E, thereby helping to arrest hardening of the arteries.

This vitamin is also considered helpful in restoring missing hair. Tests have shown that some persons have evidenced revived hair growth when they took inositol along with the other B vitamins; when the others were taken alone, however, no results were obtained.

Best natural food sources are:

beef brains	fruits	nuts
beef heart	lecithin	peas, dried
blackstrap molasses	lima beans, dry	wheat germ
brewer's yeast	liver	whole grains
cantaloupe	meat	yogurt
corn	milk, whole	

NIACIN

Niacin, well known as the substance that defends the body against pellagra, is necessary for healthy blood, fine skin tone, and sound digestion. Niacin retards the accumulation of cholesterol and other fatty substances in the bloodstream that contribute to hardening of the arteries. It is also required for good circulation, for the health of the brain and nervous system, for ideal functioning of the liver, and finally, for the combustion of starch and sugar. Unfortunately, niacin is one of the members of the B-complex that is removed from flour and sugar in the processing.

Niacin is frequently termed the "courage vitamin," because even a modest deficiency can influence the personality and bring on deviations from the norm such as apprehension, forgetfulness, hostility, insomnia, low morale, mental disturbances, surliness, suspicion, tension, and so on.

An undue scarcity of niacin causes or results in diarrhea, inflammation of the intestinal tract, severe skin disease, sore tongue and mouth, and loss of appetite, strength, and weight.

Conditions such as those just mentioned can be remedied, and especially by keeping to a diet in which brewer's yeast (which induces normal digestion and elimination), beefsteak, and liver and other meats are predominant. Other good food sources are:

barley, whole	kidney	rice polishings
chicken	lobster	soybeans
eggs	mushrooms	turkey
fish	nuts	wheat germ
heart	peanuts	whey

PANTOTHENIC ACID

For many years this vitamin of the B-complex has been designated as an antidermatitic agent, since one of its notable functions is protection of the skin. In addition, pantothenic acid is highly important to growth and helps to forestall old-age symptoms, such as impaired adrenal glands, accumulations of fat in the liver and kidneys, thinning hair, and shriveled testicles.

It favorably affects the activity of the digestive system and the entire alimentary canal and is an effective detoxifier of such body poisons as cortisone, DDT, streptomycin, strychnine, and sulfa drugs. This vitamin is also used in the treatment of neuritis and rheumatoid arthritis.

Human beings whose diet was improved with additional B vitamins exceeding ordinary requirements showed a marked increase in their resistance to mental stress. They attained a greater degree of steadiness and self-control under pressure, and pantothenic acid proved especially valuable in this connection.

This would seem to be a more sensible course to take than self-dosage with tranquilizers, don't you agree?

Good sources of this vitamin are:

beans	corn	potatoes
beef	eggs	salmon
blackstrap molasses	kidneys	soybeans
brewer's yeast	liver	wheat germ
broccoli	peanuts	
cabbage	peas	

PARA-AMINO-BENZOIC ACID

Para-amino-benzoic acid is essential for the regular functioning of the glands and is now thought to be the actual element in the B-complex that delays the appearance of gray hair. Other antigray vitamins of the B-complex are choline, inositol, and pantothenic acid. It is used to insure the reliable performance of the pituitary gland (which, in turn, favorably influences rheumatoid arthritis) and for treatment of rheumatic fever, and it is given to women to help overcome sterility. It is also administered by allergists for migraine headaches and for the relief of asthma.

Deficiency of this vitamin induces anemia, intense fatigue, skin rash, or eczema.

It is found most plentifully in:

blackstrap molasses	meat
brewer's yeast	nuts
fish	rice polishings
fruits	whole grains
liver	

VITAMIN C

Vitamin C, which is called the "master vitamin," is essential to breathing, the heartbeat, and all bodily processes. Since the body cannot manufacture its own vitamin C, one must get the needed quantities from foods or supplements; because it is a water-soluble vitamin, it must be taken daily.

Early in the nineteenth century, it was widely known that lemon juice was a safeguard against scurvy. It was not until 1932, however, that researchers and food scientists discovered and identified that unknown essence as vitamin C.

The body must have vitamin C in order to produce collagen, a sort of cement that binds the cells together. It is an essential element of connective tissue, of which it conserves the elasticity and strength. Vitamin C is called the "vitality vitamin," because it is basic to health and life; you cannot live without it. It is needed by all the glands, but it particularly encourages the production of cortisone by the adrenals. Moreover, it is an indispensable bulwark for protection against disease bacteria and maintains durability of blood-vessel walls. It is essential to health at all ages, but especially in later life.

A very large percentage of all Americans suffers to some degree from diseases of the teeth and gums. Vitamin C and its associated bioflavonoids definitely influence the health of the gums, and their condition affords a good indication of your health pattern. This substance is vital to the complete development of the teeth. If enough vitamin C is not provided to growing children, the enamel of their teeth wears away or is even lacking. Tooth cavities occur most often in children, so a generous supply of this vitamin is absolutely necessary during these years to prevent decay.

We are beset on all sides nowadays by innumerable poisons, which we cannot escape, and which take the form of chemical additives, dyes, and fertilizers. Vitamin C acts as a detoxifier of these poisons. This vitamin is also recognized to be a defensive medium in cases of asthma, eczema, hay fever, hives, poison oak and poison ivy infections, and postnasal drip. It is also effective in treating arthritis, diabetes, drug sensitivity, muscular fatigue, pernicious anemia, polio, radiation sickness, rheumatic fever, and sinus infection.

You also need vitamin C for good bone formation; to heal all types of fractures; to prevent brittle bones (if vitamin C is deficient, bones will not hold minerals); for the repair of damaged nerve tissues; and for sound gums, supple joints, and healthy arteries and veins. It has proved of real value in the relief of low back pain and spinal disc injuries.

As another of its important functions, vitamin C promotes the absorption and utilization of iron. It also acts as a mild diuretic and helps to preserve normal vision. Since it regulates the cholesterol in the bloodstream, it is an important agent in lowering high blood pressure.

Medical authorities have published impressive results of treatment with vitamin C of chicken pox, diphtheria, dysentery, influenza, measles, mumps, pelvic infections, scarlet fever, septicemia, shingles, and tuberculosis.

Prevention Magazine (September 1963) reported on a survey that pointed out that vitamin C has the astounding qualification of being able to take the place of any of the other vitamins in a crisis.

According to a study in *Clinical Medicine,* Vitamin C has been used successfully in treating the common cold.

> There have been many reports in the literature indicating that massive doses of vitamin C are of value in treating virus infections. . . . Doses as high as 10 grams (10,000 milligrams) have been administered intravenously without ill effects.[2]

In six cases of virus infections treated with vitamin C,

[2] *Health Bulletin* (July 20, 1963).

"there was prompt patient response. In four of the patients, improvement was considered dramatic."

When one considers the fact that the average adult gets four colds a year and loses eight days from his job, which costs him or his boss eight days' pay—aside from the cost of medication and doctor's bills—the magnitude of the problem can be quickly seen. Do you begin to see that there is a solution—that you can prevent colds by the use of this remarkable food?

The *Journal of the American Medical Association* referred to a British study (1963) in which saturation with ascorbic acid (vitamin C) was used as a treatment for forty male chronic psychiatric patients. Some had been in mental hospitals for as long as forty-five years. "The results showed that saturation with vitamin C has brought about an improvement in over-all personality functioning."[3] The article explained that psychiatric patients are known to have "an unusually high demand for ascorbic acid," and that the hospital catering did not meet that demand. Vitamin supplementation of the diet was recommended.

A deficiency of vitamin C causes many grievous and diversified bodily evils, not the least of which is a loss of vitalizing oxygen. A deficiency may also lead to the formation of kidney stones and to other improper usage of calcium by the body.

Vitamin C shortages can also lead to aching bones, joints and muscles, apathy, fatigue, shortness of breath, sterility, and weakness. Likewise, deficiency can worsen allergies, cause the breakdown of gum tissues, introducing

---

[3] "Ascorbic acid in chronic psychiatric patients—A controlled trial," *British Journal of Psychiatry,* March 1963 (quoted in *Journal of the American Medical Association* [Vol. 185, No. 2; July 13, 1963], 221).

pyorrhea, and cause hemorrhaging of capillaries (the smallest blood vessels).

Reports indicate that the greatest single cause of a lowered vitamin C supply in the average person is regular smoking. Tests show that the smoking of one cigarette neutralizes about twenty-five milligrams of vitamin C in the body.

The National Research Council recommends seventy-five to one hundred milligrams daily as the minimum intake to prevent scurvy, but each person must discover his own requirements, depending upon his or her own particular circumstances.

In past years, one of the scourges of my life was severe chest colds. If I happened to lose much sleep, or got wet feet, or was under tension or anxious, I would invariably come down with a cold or cough and, once it had begun, no matter what I did, I was never successful in arresting it; it always went the limit. Now I take daily an average of twelve hundred milligrams of C, combined with the bioflavonoids, and I am virtually immune to these infections. So test and study your reactions until you have found the right dosage.

Actually, as far as I know, there is no limit to the amount of natural vitamin C that one can safely take, since any excess is eliminated by the kidneys very rapidly. There is no allergic or toxic reaction from vitamin C. It is the opinion of many nutritionists that everyone should get very much more vitamin C. There is no danger of getting too much.

Practically all fresh natural foods contain vitamin C, but rose hips contain more per gram than any other food. They also contain the bioflavonoids (vitamin P) and some vitamin A. Rose hips are the fruit of the rose, which remain after the petals have fallen. Rose hips may also be obtained in convenient powder, liquid, or tablet form in health food shops. Other excellent food sources are:

apples	citrus fruits[4]	peas
apricots	collards	persimmons
asparagus	corn, sweet	pimentos
avocados	green beans	pineapple
bananas	green peppers	potatoes
beet greens	kale	sardines
berries	lima beans	soybeans
broccoli	liver	strawberries
brussels sprouts	melons	tomatoes
cabbage	parsley	turnips
cantaloupe	parsnips	watercress
cauliflower	peaches	

VITAMIN D

Vitamin D is a fat-soluble vitamin that is absolutely essential for health, and especially for that of children, since it is required for the proper use of calcium and phosphorus by the body. Both these minerals are necessary for strong bones and teeth. The available evidence is conclusive that this vitamin is indispensable for their absorption and that it promotes their efficiency. It has also been proven beyond all question that vitamin D prevents rickets.

Vitamin D is called the "sunshine vitamin," as it is produced by the action of sunlight on a substance secreted by the oil glands of the skin. It is a vital aid to the health of the nervous system: another natural tranquilizer, which relaxes the nerves and induces sound sleep.

[4] *Caution:* Citrus fruits and juices should be used very sparingly, as they cause an alkaline urine, a circumstance that is conducive to the increase of disease bacteria.

One authority writes, on the subject of synthetic vitamin D:

> Do you give your child "Viosterol" or "Vigautol" (synthetic Vitamin D)? It is well established that this product causes blood in the urine very quickly in children, by its destructive action to the kidneys. Deaths have been reported from the ordinary dosages used to "protect" from rickets.[5]

You need more vitamin D for the building of energy, for the better absorption of minerals, for eye health, regular heart action, and effective clotting of the blood. It is of the greatest importance to the health of the thyroid gland, and some kinds of arthritis have been improved and even cured by it.

It is also valuable in other respects, and has been used in treatment of lockjaw, nearsightedness, osteomalacia, osteoporosis, and psoriasis. It is especially advantageous in healing fractured bones, during pregnancy and lactation, and again throughout the course of the menopause. If coupled with calcium, it is also useful for prevention of despondency, hot flashes, irritation, muscle spasms, and night sweats. As one advances in age, one's need for this vitamin increases.

An insufficiency of vitamin D prevents the body from using sugar efficiently, so that fatigue results. Other conditions caused by a deficiency of this vitamin are arthritis, defective teeth, imperfect bone structure, softening of the bones (osteomalacia), and nervous tension.

Speaking of sunshine in connection with vitamin D, a doctor in Arizona, where I was living, once told me that the time one was exposed to sunlight while going to and from work each day was enough to provide one with his

[5] Richard D. Townsend, *Let's Talk Health Sense* (Boston: Bruce, Humphries, 1960).

daily quota of vitamin D. At the time, I made a practice of sitting out in the sun in a park near my home for a couple of hours nearly every day. The doctor forbade this, saying that it raised the temperature of the body, which was dangerous. I have followed that advice ever since; but, realizing that vitamin D is relatively scarce in foods, I take an additional supplement of 3,500 units a day.

The National Research Council recommends only four hundred units of vitamin D daily for individuals of all ages. Medical studies disclose, however, that about four thousand units can be taken every day to advantage, because this vitamin is not plentiful in ordinary foods.

Cod liver oil, halibut liver oil, and other fish liver oils are the only satisfactory food sources. Other foods that have some vitamin D are:

butter	oysters
eggs	salmon
herring	sardines
liver	sunflower seeds
mackerel	tunafish
milk	

For quite a while I have been using a halibut liver oil capsule, which provides 850 units of vitamin D and five thousand units of vitamin A. It has proved to be very satisfactory. Make sure to obtain this vitamin from a natural source.

VITAMIN E

Vitamin E is really a fat-soluble group, the elements of which are designated alpha, beta, gamma, and delta (the first four letters of the Greek alphabet). At present, however, according to the best available authorities, the only active member of the group is the alpha ingredient.

When the millers began the custom of separating the wheat germ from the substance of the kernel, the principal source of vitamin E was milled out of the flour, so that now it cannot be obtained from bread or other white-flour products. As a result of this practice, a decline in public health began. Consequently, there is an unusual amount of general interest in the use of vitamin E, which is essential for normal functioning of the cardiovascular system.

If you use white flour and its products, you are certainly deficient in vitamin E, because this substance is chiefly found in whole grains. I believe that the American diet does not contain enough vitamin E for good health. All the evidence points in that direction.

> The veterinarians have known for forty years that vitamin E is also necessary for normal reproduction. They have given wheat germ oil to the barren heifers and to the bulls, with good results.
> I am convinced that vitamin E is also necessary for normal reproduction in humans. I believe that one of the reasons why young women have so many menstrual disorders, and one of the reasons why they are having more miscarriages and so much more trouble at the menopause, is because our modern diet has been robbed of its vitamin E.[6]

Vitamin E is essential for everyone from infancy to old age. It is especially needed by young people and by all who make vigorous demands upon the heart. It is one of the major foods of the pituitary gland, the adrenals, and the

[6] Statement of Dr. J. Nichols, President of Natural Food Associates, quoted in Cathryn Elwood, *Feel Like a Million* (New York: Devin-Adair Co., 1958).

sex glands. It is also important in that it helps the liver to detoxify various injurious substances and stave off many diseases of the later years.

Vitamin E is prescribed by physicians for men who have withered testicles. In this connection, I should mention that it is a known fact that this element is effective in influencing the youthfulness of the sex glands and prolonging their normal activity. Understanding the relation of nutrition to marital happiness can be an important step toward removing what may be the underlying cause of much incompatibility in married life.

Far better than drugs, vitamin E serves as an anticoagulant, dilates the blood vessels, and prevents blood clots from forming in the arteries, capillaries, and veins. No known food element has such a multiplicity of healing qualities as vitamin E. It is truly unique.

The body has more call for vitamin E in the cells and tissues than any other food, and it is second to none in its curative power. The healing of bruises, burns, and wounds is speeded up by the action of vitamin E; it prevents the formation of too much scar tissue, and sometimes even melts scar tissue that is incidental in urinary tract strictures.

This important substance was discovered in 1922 by researchers at the Universities of Arkansas and California. Since then it has been used successfully to ease the following conditions:

acne	diabetes	osteomyelitis
angina pectoris	gangrene	painful breasts
apoplexy	headaches	peptic ulcer
asthma	hot flashes	phlebitis
Berger's disease	indolent ulcer	rheumatic heart
brittle bones	kidney disease	disease
cataract	menopause distress	urethral stricture
chickenpox scars	muscular dystrophy	varicose veins

Vitamin E is usually referred to by nutritionists as the chief heart food, since its inclusion in the diet prevents degeneration of the muscles. Muscles famished for this food element need several times the quantity of oxygen that healthy muscles do. Vitamin E has a singular influence on the effective activity of all the muscles, and indications are that it is of importance in producing muscle power and preserving muscle tone. It has also been found effective in relieving the pain of muscular inflammation.

The next most important effect of the use of vitamin E is oxygen conservation. It oxygenates the tissues in the same way in which exercise invigorates. The amount of oxygen in the blood is vital, not only for the protection of a healthy body, but also for the rebuilding of injured and unhealthy tissues. Vitamin E reduces the oxygen requirement in tissues, thereby protecting the brain, heart, and kidneys.

Its ability to conserve oxygen renders it very helpful in preventing arteriosclerosis, coronary and cerebral thrombosis, congenital heart disease, diabetes, gangrene, Raynaud's syndrome, and strokes. A shortage of oxygen in the blood is a significant factor in provoking a heart attack. Due to its power to buttress capillary walls, it can ease pain of nephritis (Bright's disease), rheumatic fever, and strictures.

By keeping the oxygen supply up, vitamin E makes it possible for the body to function normally, to avoid illness, to get along on less oxygen, and build up a reserve for future needs. The benefits derived extend from better mental efficiency to unusual physical stamina, less heart stress, and improved alertness. An all-round wonderful food substance indeed!

Without additional wheat germ, or capsules of concentrated vitamin E, the average American diet probably contains a daily maximum of from twelve to fifteen international units of this substance, an amount grossly insufficient to maintain the health and strength of the cardiovascular system. Most authorities on this subject have estimated that one needs a minimum intake of thirty units a day for adequate protection. Here again it should be stressed that one must find one's own proper dosage by experimenting. I began with one hundred units a day. The first unexpected result I obtained from this food was the healing, in about six weeks, of several lesions I had had for several years on both my legs below the knees. I then increased my intake to two hundred units a day for the next thirty days, then to three hundred units for the following thirty days, and so on until I built my consumption up to six hundred units a day, which I found to be the most effective dose for me. I have been taking this amount for about eight years with excellent results.

In view of the scarcity of vitamin E in the average diet, an eminent medical authority wrote that everyone should be taking daily supplements of natural vitamin E. I say "natural," because it has been ascertained that the natural form of this vitamin is five times as potent as the synthetic product.

Foods in which vitamin E is most plentiful are:

apples	haddock	pork chops
avocados	kale	rice, brown
bacon	kelp	sardines
bananas	lamb chops	seeds
barley	lettuce	soybean oil
beefsteak	liver	sunflower seed oil
butter	olive oil	sweet potatoes
carrots	onions	tomatoes
coconut oil	parsley	turnip greens
corn oil	peanut oil	wheat germ
cottonseed oil	peas	wheat germ oil
eggs	potatoes	whole grains

—And, of course, capsules of concentrated vitamin E, since it is practically impossible to get enough of this vitamin without resorting to fresh vegetable oils or concentrates for your daily needs.

Note: The need for vitamin E increases as the intake of polyunsaturated fats rises.

VITAMIN F (UNSATURATED FATTY ACIDS)

Fats are one of the three main building substances necessary for maintaining life. They are the most condensed form of energy and, consequently, even very small amounts of them will serve.

Vitamin F (the unsaturated fatty acids) is necessary for general good health, attractive skin, and quiet nerves. It helps in the absorption of the fat-soluble vitamins A, D, E, and K, as well as assisting in distributing calcium to the tissues. Certain exceptional growth elements are contained in it.

Medical evidence indicates that vitamin F is useful in the successful treatment of prostate gland trouble. Cases treated experienced a rapid decrease in swelling. It is also given credit for emulsifying cholesterol in the bloodstream, making it harmless. It likewise helps to make the joints more pliable.

Vitamin F is salutary in decreasing the number of colds one gets and reduces their severity; so that, on this account alone, this substance is a very desirable addition to the diet. These acids also aid the reproductive processes and are believed to have some connection with the proper operation of the thyroid gland. An active thyroid fosters an attractive, graceful body.

I have used several vegetable oils for varying periods

of time, but, so far as benefits to the skin are concerned, I got the best results with corn oil. Corn oil contains the following acids, all important to health: arachidic, lignoceric, linoleic (an ingredient indispensable to life itself), linolenic, oleic, palmitric, and stearic. Many sufferers from arthritis, asthma, dandruff, fatigue, kidney disease, leg pains, migraine headache, psoriasis, eczema, and other skin diseases have responded to this therapy. Deficiencies of vitamin F can be responsible for brittle and lusterless hair and nails and dry skin.

In conclusion, a word about wheat germ oil. This valuable oil furnishes energy and vitality and helps the body to cope with the saturated fats. It has been proven to increase endurance. Progress was made and symptoms suppressed in some people with progressive muscular dystrophy and neuromuscular disorders who received wheat germ oil.

Dr. T. K. Cureton, head of the University of Illinois Physical Fitness Laboratory, said that wheat germ oil helps men to do hard labor without harm and to withstand severe stress. It increases stamina.

Vitamin F is found particularly in cereal and vegetable oils, as well as seed fats. The following foods are the best sources:

corn oil	soybean oil
cottonseed oil	sunflower seeds and oil
peanuts and peanut oil	wheat germ oil
safflower oil	whole grains
sesame seeds and oil	

VITAMIN K

Vitamin K is the blood-clotting food element. It stops hemorrhaging following bodily injury, childbirth, a tooth extraction, or surgery. Its best food source is leafy greens.

VITAMIN P (THE BIOFLAVONOIDS)

Vitamin P (the bioflavonoids) is an aggregate of citrin, hesperidin, and rutin. It is present mainly in the pulpy portion of fruits and other fresh foods, always accompanied by vitamin C. For this reason, the effectiveness of vitamins P and C is greatly reinforced when they act as a team, more so than if they are taken individually.

Since vitamin P promotes ideal capillary penetration, it is of importance in keeping the heart and blood vessel walls in good, healthy condition. The action of this food benefits such grave conditions as arteriosclerosis, coronary thrombosis, and hemorrhaging. It likewise minimizes the risk of strokes and helps prevent the familiar degenerative conditions we see all around us today.

Vitamin P acts favorably on the tiniest veins, the capillaries, through which all nutrients pass from the blood into the cells and tissues and waste material is gathered and removed from the body. In this manner it accomplishes wonders in aiding all kinds of afflictions by stimulating basic body resistance against attack.

You also need vitamin P for protection against a number of ailments, including: bursitis, cirrhosis of the liver, diabetes, eczema, glaucoma, high blood pressure, miscarriage, polio, psoriasis, rheumatic fever, and rheumatoid arthritis. Combined with vitamin C, it has also proved beneficial in respiratory infections, from the well-known cold to influenza, tonsillitis, and tuberculosis.

Foods that are especially rich in this wonder-working substance are:

currants, black and red	parsley
citrus fruits	prunes
grapes	rose hips
green peppers	spinach

Next best sources are:

apples	lettuce	sweet potatoes
apricots	parsnips	tomatoes
cabbage	peas	walnuts
carrots	plums	watercress
cherries	potatoes	

Before entering into a detailed explanation of the various minerals and their functions in the body, I feel it will be helpful to pause a few moments in order to summarize briefly some of the important points covered in this section on the vitamins.

To obtain the vitamins outlined in the preceding pages in maximum quantity and optimum quality, eat the following foods, which supply these nutrients in their most concentrated form:

FOR VITAMIN A

A basic high-protein diet, including green and yellow fruits and vegetables, butter, and fish liver oil perles or cod liver oil

FOR VITAMIN B-COMPLEX

A basic high-protein diet, supplemented with brewer's yeast, desiccated liver, peanuts, sesame seeds, sunflower seeds, and yogurt

FOR VITAMIN C

Fresh green vegetables, fresh raw fruits, melons, raw and canned tomatoes and tomato juice, and strawberries, supplemented with rose-hip preparations

FOR VITAMIN D

Egg yolk, fish and fish liver oils, milk and milk products, oysters, sardines, and sunflower seeds

FOR VITAMIN E

Eggs, fish, liver, vegetable oils, wheat germ and wheat germ oil, and vitamin E capsules

FOR VITAMIN F

Corn oil, lecithin granules, nuts, safflower oil, sesame oil, soybean oil, sunflower oil and seeds, and wheat germ oil

FOR VITAMIN P

Black and red currants, citrus fruits, grapes, green peppers, parsley, prunes, spinach, cabbage, carrots, peas, potatoes, sweet potatoes, tomatoes, and walnuts, supplemented with rose-hip preparations

5

MINERALS—POWER TO SPARE

WE are all very much alike in that we want uninterrupted good health, along with the vitality and stamina to enjoy our work or play; but protein, carbohydrates, and fats alone are not enough to assure us of these physical blessings. The body also requires special substances known as minerals. If minerals are lacking, the vitamins cannot perform their various functions; if vitamins are absent, however, the body can make some use of minerals.

As with vitamins, the body needs ever so little of each of the minerals, but minerals in their proper balance can make the difference between illness and glowing health.

The body needs at least sixteen minerals to maintain energy and lengthen life, and I believe that the minerals are very much more important to health than most people realize. Somewhere along the line, the fact that the content of the human body is a mineral one has been forgotten, even though this basic truth is mentioned in the Book of Genesis.

Minerals are able to maintain the water balance in your body which [is] required for life processes. They draw chemical substances in and out of your cells. Minerals help to keep blood and tissue fluid from becoming either too acid or too alkaline. Minerals also stimulate glandular secretion of hormones and influence the nervous system which sends mental messages throughout all of your body organs, limbs, etc. Minerals are able to nourish your body to prevent irritability and help in the contractibility of muscles.*

We must supply minerals to the body daily, as they are vitally necessary to conserve and help recondition blood, bones, brains, hair, heart, muscles, nerves, and teeth. All of them are imperative to gland functions. They are also required for the development, health, vigor, and efficient operation of many other parts of the body. They are essential for adequate blood circulation as well as for good heart and blood vessel tone.

Since healthy blood needs to be more alkaline than acid, minerals are needed in order to perform this delicate balance by adding proper amounts of copper and iron.

When mineral deficiences accumulate, the bones become brittle and break easily, teeth go bad, and brain cells and the heart muscle do not perform their functions properly. Unless there is a constant daily intake, the blood will withdraw minerals from the tissues and bones. It was not realized until recently that mineral deficiencies also caused a depletion of strength and virility.

The average American's diet is nearly always meagerly supplied with minerals, due to the widespread processing of foodstuffs. Therefore, you must be sure to eat foods containing calcium, iron, phosphorus, potassium, and sulphur. Trace minerals, such as iodine, nickel, and silver, are also being more and more generally acclaimed for the important services they render the body.

* All quotations in Chapter 5 are from *Health Saver* Magazine (Vol. 5, No. 1; 1962).

CALCIUM

Minerals, in truth, are integral parts of all the bones and tissues, and the absolutely supreme mineral in the human body, on a quantitative basis, is calcium. It is a metallic element usually found in nature in association with other chemicals. Its efficacy in the body is regulated by two pairs of very small glands called parathyroids. Your bones are more than two thirds mineral content, and the dominant mineral is calcium. Calcium gives solidity to bones and teeth, and in order to lengthen life it is important that you fortify your bones.

Calcium is the most abundant mineral in your body; it comprises more than 2% of your weight. About 99% of this calcium is stored in your bones and teeth. A mere 1% then circulates throughout all the soft tissues and body fluids. This mineral is needed for healing of wounds, blood clotting, for the stimulation of certain enzyme action and to control the passage of fluid through the cell and tissue walls. The proper amount of calcium in your blood is needed for the alternate contraction and relaxation of the heart muscles.

Just as vitamin C is the key vitamin, so calcium could be termed the key mineral. When there is too little calcium in the bloodstream, the body develops a kind of undernourishment, which is damaging to bones, heart, muscles, nerves, and teeth—the health of which is the origin of a vigorous body and mind. Every muscle in the body, including the heart, relies on calcium for its power, and the heart cannot relax if calcium is at a low ebb.

The need for calcium is continuous throughout life, and it is well-known that the body demands calcium as

it does no other single factor. It is one of the most vital
nutritional elements required for the formation and rebuilding of body tissues. Growing children especially need
a liberal amount of calcium when bones and teeth are
developing. Likewise, pregnant women and nursing mothers need additional calcium. It strengthens and regulates
the heart, preserves powerful muscular elasticity, and induces sound sleep. Spasms in the intestine, usually referred to as colitis, or spastic constipation, are generally
alleviated by ample amounts of this mineral. A liberal
intake is usually followed by better body development,
while at the same time it helps steady nerves and relieve
exhausting tensions.

Calcium has been found to be very useful as a pain
reliever, regardless of the cause of the pain. For instance,
it is alleged that migraine headache sufferers can often
obtain relief by taking calcium. It is also said that calcium will soothe the pain of arthritis in from one to three
days. Likewise, nutritionists advise that an increased
amount be taken during menstrual periods and throughout the course of the menopause.

It is not widely known that the absorption of calcium
is blocked by many drugs and some foods, such as bread,
chocolate, and cocoa; it is interfered with by anything
that encourages the flow of alkaline gastric juices. Sodium
fluoride, which has been added to drinking water in many
communities, also produces such a result.

The inability to utilize calcium effectively is widespread, regardless of the fact that this mineral is so essential to health and especially critical to the well-being of
middle-aged and older persons.

While only 1 percent of the calcium intake is used by
the soft tissues, if the body does not obtain it the sub-
sequent signs readily appear: bad posture, brittle bones,
cramps in the abdomen and legs, nervous tension, rapid

heartbeat (often linked with nervousness), receding of bone around the teeth, and tooth decay. Loss of this vital substance is the main cause of osteoporosis and bone frailty. This is clearly indicated in the case of many elderly people, whose bones may be broken with very little force, as well as in the frequency with which cataracts form during the later years.

According to some medical authorities, the American dietary is perhaps more lacking in calcium than in any other essential food. Calcium deficiency is one of the known causes of premature aging. Dr. Henry C. Sherman of Columbia University, a noted biochemist, has stated:

> The prime period of human life could be extended by a moderate increase in calcium in the diet of those in or approaching the ranks of senior citizens, plus eating twice the minimum amount of protein, and a sizable increase in the daily intake of Vitamins A and C.

The National Research Council recommends that adults obtain a minimum of one thousand milligrams (one gram) each day. The same amount is recommended for growing children.

There are many excellent sources of calcium. Nearly all fresh foods contain some calcium. (Unfortunately, pasteurized milk is not a good source of this mineral.) Foods that you can count on for important amounts of calcium are:

almonds	fish	poultry
blackstrap molasses	fruits, fresh	potatoes
broccoli	honey	sprouts
buttermilk	kale	soybeans
cheese	meat	turnip greens
collards	mustard greens	whole grains
cottage cheese	nuts	yogurt
eggs		

The very best supplementary source of calcium is bone meal. Other supplementary sources are calcium gluconate, calcium lactate, calcium tablets, and sea kelp.

CHLORINE

This mineral acts as a cleanser of the body. As it naturally appears in food, it is useful in producing hydrochloric acid in the stomach.

Here is a mineral which acts like the broomstick of nature by removing toxic waste products from your system. Chlorine stimulates production of hydrochloric acid in the digestive tract so that proteins may be properly worked upon and utilized. Chlorine is helpful to keep a supple joint and tendon condition and has been seen to distribute the hormones secreted by your endocrine glands.

Shortage of chlorine can hamper growth and cause anxiety and uneasiness.

Best food sources are: beets, leafy greens, milk, radishes, raw meat, ripe olives, and table salt.

COPPER

Copper is necessary for the proper use of iron by the body and is therefore of importance in preventing anemia. This mineral has something to do with pigment composition and may have an influence in preserving hair color. Copper also aids bone marrow in the production of red blood cells. With iodine and iron, this substance is necessary for healthy sex glands.

This essential mineral combines with iron to help metabolize food into hemoglobin, the oxygen-carrying substance found within the red blood cells. Copper is also needed by stomach enzymes for proper function. Copper is also found in the liver, bile, blood, and is required for the assimilation of iron. . . . The formation of melanin, the pigment of the skin, also depends on this essential mineral, [which] also aids in utilization of vitamin C.

Lack of copper results in impaired breathing and habitual weakness.

Copper is usually well supplied in good, natural foods; reliable sources are:

almonds	egg yolk	prunes
apricots	figs	shrimp
beans, dried	liver	soy flour
blackstrap molasses	loganberries	vegetables, green
clams	oysters	whole grains

IODINE

Iodine is one of the so-called trace minerals, of which the body requires only a very minute quantity. What is a trace? One one thousandth of an ounce for an adult; but this trifling pittance is sufficient for the body's needs, and you must have it—or die! Iodine is located almost entirely in the thyroid gland, and is necessary for the proper functioning of that gland.

You need iodine to relieve nervous tension, for greater endurance and stamina, and for controlling weight. It is especially required by the thyroid gland to produce the hormone thyroxin, which promotes growth and is an important factor in the conservation of health from top to toe.

Iodine cooperates with iron in the body and reacts favorably upon sexual potency. The blood vessels, brain, and heart and the endocrine system share the benefits derived from iodine-rich foods.

Women should have more iodine and iron because their losses of these nutrients through menstruation, gestation, and lactation are quite considerable. Iodine is further required for the digestion, assimilation and combustion of fats.

A deficiency of iodine may cause goiter, an enlarged neck. It may also lead to myxedema—complete cessation of the secretion of the thyroid—which causes overweight, sluggishness, and lowered mentality.

The major source of iodine is the ocean. Animal and plant foods from the ocean are a trustworthy source of iodine. Two superior iodine-rich seafoods are haddock and codfish. Cod liver oil is also a long-accepted and approved source. Clams, lobsters, and oysters are other good iodine foods. In addition, dehydrated sea vegetation, such as dulse and kelp, are first-class sources of the highest quality. Garlic is the best vegetable source.

Other food sources are:

asparagus	lettuce	potatoes
bananas	milk	radishes
cabbage	milk products	salmon
carrots	mushrooms	seeds
celery	onions	strawberries
egg yolk	peanuts	tomatoes
fruits	peas	tunafish

In many cases, taking an undue amount of iodine will neither increase nor decrease thyroid gland activity. If you are eating a good diet containing some of the foods suggested above, you are no doubt obtaining enough iodine. Remember—the body needs only a trace!

IRON

Iron is present to some extent in most natural foods, and this important mineral is in certain respects the most significant of the mineral family, not only because it is important in building energy, but because it prevents anemia.

Iron is necessary for good, healthy blood, which conveys blood sugar, food, oxygen, and other nutrients to all parts of the body.

Throughout the billions of body cells and tissues in your system, each tiny one must depend upon iron for a supply of oxygen—its breath of life. Your brain requires oxygen for proper function and iron is needed to carry oxygen throughout your body to all blood capillaries and tissues, including those located in your brain. Poor heart beat, a bluish-white eyeball condition, poor skin health may be traced to an iron-poor diet.

Anemia is one of the most treacherous diseases known. It subtly saps the foundation of resistance, allowing infection to invade the body. Further, anemia can induce dull, prematurely gray hair, untimely wrinkling of the skin, fingernails that break easily, shortness of breath, and a raw, inflamed mouth and tongue. It is estimated by many nutritionists that approximately 90 percent of American women are afflicted with anemia to some degree. Moreover, anemia can lead to mental derangement occurring in association with excessive disappointment and worry over lack of success or an unfavorable situation.

Due to the discovery of vitamin B-12, fortunately, pernicious anemia seems to be under control now. Minute doses of B-12 are much more powerful than liver alone, and prospects of relief from this serious disease are favorable.

A diet adequate in protein and the B-complex vitamins from natural sources will ordinarily be well supplied with iron.

The National Research Council's usual recommendation is at least twelve milligrams of iron daily for a man, and fifteen milligrams for a woman: more if the menstrual flow is profuse and during pregnancy and lactation.

The following foods are good sources:

apricots (best fruit source)	kidney
	lamb
barley, whole	liver
beef	oysters
blackstrap molasses	peanuts
brewer's yeast	prunes
clams	raisins
egg yolk	tongue
green vegetables (parsley is the richest source)	turkey (best meat source)
heart	wheat germ
honey	whole grains

MAGNESIUM

Another fundamental body mineral is magnesium. So vital is it to your welfare that an adequate or inadequate intake can mean the difference between health and disease. It is required for normal muscle activity and has a bearing on the action of enzymes in the body.

Magnesium is closely related to both calcium and phosphorus in its location and its functions in the body. About 70% of the magnesium in the body is in the bones. The rest is in the soft tissues and blood. Magnesium acts as a starter for some of the chemical reactions within the body. It plays an important role as a co-enzyme in the building of protein. We have also noted that magnesium is nature's way to calm and cool the nervous system. This mineral also adds firmness to your bones and takes part in the formation of the albumen of the blood.

In recent years it has been brought to light (*Prevention* Magazine, December 1963) that, as far back as 1930, two French doctors obtained effective results in the treatment of urinary conditions with magnesium chloride. They found that it prevents gall bladder and kidney stones.

In 1932, Dr. Schrumpf-Pierron, Professor of Medicine at the Sorbonne in Paris, studied the health of thirteen million Egyptians and concluded that magnesium in their diet is a cancer preventative. This was confirmed by Dr. Pierre Delbet of the French Academy of Medicine in 1944, after exhaustive soil and crop analyses and statistical studies.

Additionally, magnesium has been found to be the most effective single ingredient in promoting good bone structure. It is an efficient agent against pyorrhea, as it aids the assimilation of other minerals and restores natural bone solidity. It also benefits degenerative artery disorders and causes excessive calcium and osteophytes (hardened swellings on a tendon or bone) to disappear. It is even reported effective against ordinary body odors.

In some unknown way it suppresses substances in waste that cause odor.

Deficiency of magnesium causes a disturbance of the calcification of the bone. A scarcity of this mineral is also detrimental to the blood vessels, the blood pressure, and the heart, and is a significant factor in causing periodontal disease, osteoporosis, and even epilepsy. Believe it or not, many children classed as dull or backward are often merely deficient in magnesium. This raises the interesting possibility that "problem children" may be undernourished.

Magnesium is abundant in green leaves. Seeds and nuts are also known to be high in magnesium content. You can protect yourself against a deficit by using any of the following foods:

almonds	corn	peas, dried
beet greens	endive	pecans
blackstrap molasses	hazelnuts	pumpkin seeds
bone meal	honey	soy flour
brazil nuts	kelp	sunflower seeds
buckwheat, whole	kohlrabi	walnuts
grain	lima beans, dried	wheat germ
cashew nuts	peanuts	

As a supplement to the above foods, a new product is now available in health food and diet shops, in convenient tablet form, under the trade name Dolomite. This is a combination of natural sources of magnesium and calcium, with the emphasis on magnesium.

The recommended quantity of magnesium to take daily is seven to ten milligrams per kilogram of body weight, or approximately 448 to 640 milligrams. I use eight Dolomite tablets a day, which yield about 625 milligrams. The average American's intake is less than three hundred milligrams per day. Because the body excretes magnesium quickly, it should be taken several times a day.

PHOSPHORUS

Phosphorus serves as a solidifying agent in building bones and teeth and makes them strong. In the tissues it combines with the very essence of each cell. This mineral directly affects the brain cells, sustaining the appropriate fluid content, and, in union with calcium, it reinforces the functions and power of the brain, nerves, and muscles.

Phosphorus is needed as well to stabilize the acid-alkaline level in the blood and urine, for all glandular secretions, for muscle contraction, and for that vital spark. It also stimulates enzymes and assists in the digestion of carbohydrates and fats.

This mineral combines with calcium; for utilization, each requires the presence of the other. Phosphorus blends with calcium for ossification or calcification to create strong bones. Phosphorus is an essential constituent of every living body tissue. It takes part in the chemical reactions with proteins, fats and carbohydrates to produce body energy to stimulate growth and repair. It helps your blood to neutralize excess acidity and maintain a healthy alkaline condition.

Deficiency of phosphorus results in brittle bones, faulty appetite, rickets, sluggish growth, tendency to pyorrhea, tooth decay, weakness, and weight loss.

All protein foods, like cheese, eggs, fish, meats, and nuts, and nearly all vegetables and fruits contain some phosphorus. Other good sources are:

beet tops	red cabbage
cranberries	soybeans
poultry	whole grains

Remember: Calcium and phosphorus are assimilated in the body only when vitamin D is present.

POTASSIUM

Potassium is to the heart and nerves what calcium is to the bones. One should not neglect this mineral in view of its necessity for the harmonious functioning of the nervous system and the building and conserving of body resources. There is no substitute.

One of its principal tasks is to maintain the suppleness and pliability of the tissues. It is one of the most vital of all the minerals, being necessary for consistent development of the body; there can be no life without it. This mineral inhibits the thickening that threatens the entire cardiovascular system. Vigor, muscular endurance, and normal blood pressure are only three of the substantial physical gains to be expected from the extraordinary mineral potassium.

This mineral joins with phosphorus to cause oxygen to be transported to the cells of your brain. It also nourishes the muscular system and aids in normalization of the heart beat. You need potassium to invigorate your kidney to aid in disposing of body waste products and also for muscular contraction strength. Your entire glandular and hormonal systems are influenced by potassium.

In addition, potassium conserves body fluids and assists in the utilization of protein. It is also resorted to in the treatment of dizziness, fatigue, chronic headache (including migraine), high blood pressure, and overweight, and it has been of great value in controlling diarrhea.

A lack of this mineral produces conditions favorable to constipation, indigestion, insomnia, loss of mental agility, muscular fatigue, nervousness, pimples, retarded growth, spasms in body muscles, and proneness to colds, and can lead ultimately to congestive heart failure.

To obtain plenty of potassium, use the following foods:

almonds	cherries	lentils
apple cider vinegar	cucumbers	olives
apple juice	figs	onions
blackberries	fruits	potatoes
blackstrap molasses	grape juice	prunes
cabbage	green vegetables	tomatoes
carrots	honey	watercress
cranberry juice	kelp	whole grains

SILICON

Silicon is required for good skin, sound teeth, and tough bones. It is a constituent of albumin, blood, hair, nails, nerves, and teeth.

A lack of silicon in the diet leads to loss of hair, a pronounced decline in resistance to infection, and prompt decay of teeth.

Skin flabbiness and eyes that are dull, lustreless and drowsy may often be traced to a silicon deficiency. This mineral is found in your muscles, hair, nails, pancreas, cellular walls and all connective tissues. It joins with flourine to form tooth enamel and to build strong bones.

Good sources are:

apple cider vinegar	honey
brewer's yeast	kelp
eggs	meats
fish	nuts
fruits	sunflower seeds
green beans	

SULPHUR

Sulphur purifies and tones up the blood, and has been credited with being the "beauty mineral," because it is needed for healthy hair, nails, and skin. It helps the liver to assimilate minerals and encourages the secretion of bile.

Sulphur strengthens your blood stream and renders it more powerful to resist bacterial infection. . . . A deficiency of sulphur may be noted by acne and poor hair and nail health.

Protein foods and the following vegetables and nuts contain sulphur:

almonds	figs	kohlrabi
brussel sprouts	garlic	mustard greens
cabbage	hazelnuts	peaches
carrots	honey	pecans
eggs	kale	radishes

ZINC

The human body in good health contains more zinc than any other mineral. Zinc is present in all tissues, and is mostly localized in the thyroid gland. It is believed to be required for the effective action of vitamins B-1 (thiamine) and B-12. Moreover, it is known to be an ingredient of several enzymes in the body and also functions as an energy producer.

This mineral, not too widely known, is a vital food substance. It joins with phosphorus to improve brain health via the tissues. It is believed to stimulate action of vitamins. In particular, it aids in tissue respiration— the intake of oxygen and expulsion of carbon dioxide and toxic wastes. Insulin, the hormone, depends upon zinc for proper utilization. Zinc, too, is involved in the utilization of carbohydrates which produce body energy.

Finally, it appears to have some connection with the health of the prostate gland.

TRACE MINERALS

In addition to iodine, which has been discussed, the body requires the following trace minerals:

> boron
> bromine
> cobalt
> fluorine
> manganese
> nickel
> silver

They all influence the regulation of cells, the composition of the blood, and mental vigor, and are necessary for the reproductive functions and for growth. In general, they promote beauty and long life.

These minerals are present in:

beets	honey	mushrooms
carrots	lentils	nuts
eggs	liver	peas
fish	lobster	tomatoes
fruits	meats	whole grains
green beans		

The principal nutritional flaw in the diets of mature and older persons is a lack of protein, iron, and calcium in sufficient amounts. A review of this mineral section will clearly indicate that to obtain these nutrients a high-protein diet is a must.

For calcium, then, one should include in the diet bone meal, green leafy vegetables, potatoes, and yogurt. *For iron,* blackstrap molasses, brewer's yeast, liver, and wheat germ. *For other minerals,* blackstrap molasses, bone meal, eggs, honey, kelp tablets, liver, and seafoods.

6

SOME EXTRAORDINARY FOODS

THERE are seven unique foods that deserve special examination, study, and use, because of their great value in supplying concentrated nourishment of the best quality to the body. They are: apple cider vinegar, bone meal, brewer's yeast, lecithin, sea kelp, sunflower seeds, and yogurt.

APPLE CIDER VINEGAR

It is useful to know what apple cider vinegar can do for you, since it is a valuable food for rebuilding the body, especially during middle age and later.

To begin with, apple cider vinegar will render ineffective disease bacteria in the alimentary tract. It helps control the intestinal flora and is invaluable in improving disorders of this part of the body. Failure to obtain the acids found in this food, with the accompanying minerals, often results in illness.

Unfortunately, it is commonly assumed that one can eradicate any sickness by the expenditure of substantial amounts of money; that unless a therapy is intricate and costly, it cannot be any good. Experience has shown me that some things costing practically nothing can do wonders, and apple cider vinegar is one of those things. This simple remedy has proved powerful against many stubborn disorders. In my own case, for example, after I had been taking two teaspoonfuls in a glass of water once a day for several months, I not only felt better, but I also noticed an unexpected side effect.

I had suffered from a chronic ear infection for twenty-eight years and had despaired of ever getting rid of the trouble. Then, one morning, I observed that the infection was drying up, and shortly thereafter it ceased entirely. That was nine years ago, and I have not had a sign of ear infection since. Although I had had medical treatment for this condition for months at a time (on two occasions by a leading ear specialist), nothing helped very much until I began to use the vinegar.

Physiology textbooks tell us that the body produces a new bloodstream every twenty-eight days. The blood is slightly alkaline, but if its alkalinity is raised above ordinary levels, calcium will be deposited in the tissues. By taking a simple acid like apple cider vinegar, calcium deposits in the blood vessel walls can be prevented.

Alkaline fluids condense body liquids and interfere with good circulation, while on the other hand, acid helps to keep the blood thin. A constant state of alkalinity can contribute to cancer.

It is obvious, then, that the composition of the blood is not the result of chance, but is determined by the food and drink you assimilate, which forms the bone marrow where red blood cells are prepared.

Apple cider vinegar normalizes and improves metabolism: that is to say, it invigorates the kidneys, to help them drive out poisons and infections. It is instrumental in the proper oxidation of the blood, prevents loss of blood from the body, and tenderizes the tissues. It improves digestion and bowel action. The regular use of this acid will benefit or completely cure muscle cramps.

It is also one of the best and safest correctives for obesity. As a remedy for excess weight, apple cider vinegar, in its influence upon the metabolic processes of the body, helps in the natural assimilation of carbohydrates, so that they will give energy where otherwise they would simply produce fat.

Other conditions for which benefits are to be derived from the use of apple cider vinegar are bleeding hemorrhoids, chronic headache, dizziness, high blood pressure, nose bleeding, deposits of tartar on the teeth, sore throat, and pyelitis (inflammation in the kidneys). The inclination to bleed is lessened or prevented when an acid like apple cider vinegar is taken, because it changes an alkaline urine to one with the normal acid reaction.

Apple cider vinegar contains the following minerals: calcium, chlorine, fluorine, iron, magnesium, phosphorus, potassium, silicon, sodium, sulphur, and many trace minerals.

BONE MEAL

As stated previously, an extremely important share of the nutrients in the diet comes from the mineral family. A deficiency of calcium, phosphorus, iron, and other elements is one of the most serious nutritional problems, causing tooth decay and a great many illnesses. Bone meal is an ideal, completely balanced source of these minerals in precisely the ratio in which they are found in nature.

Bone meal is simply the powdered bones of young beef cattle, nothing more, nothing less. This extraordinary source of minerals aids digestion, facilitates the union of fractures, gives strength to the bony framework of the body, improves blood health, prevents tooth cavities, fosters healthy nerves, regulates heart action, tightens loose teeth, and is recommended for canker sores, growing pains, and pregnancy complications.

Brittle and frail bones are one of the most familiar symptoms of aging, as well as one of the most distressing conditions for those so afflicted. I have seen many cases of elderly people who have fractured an arm or a leg or a hip, usually as the consequence of a fall, and are confined to a hospital or a home for months waiting for the prolonged healing process to end.

Another common infirmity of the bones is known as osteoporosis, an undue porosity and fragility of the bone tissue, which is caused by a loss of calcium. Here is where bone meal, in which calcium and phosphorus are associated with all the trace minerals, proves of inestimable value in rebuilding the bones to normal denseness and weight.

Be it noted at this point that bone meal is not a medicine, in the usual sense of the word. For many centuries bones were made use of by our forefathers as an important food; and, in many parts of the world today, bones are eaten regularly, right along with other foods.

Some leading nutritionists declare that the body requires five grams (five thousand milligrams) of calcium a day. Growing children need more than adults. A quart of milk supplies only one gram. If you happen to be allergic to milk, or dislike drinking it, bone meal will supply this indispensable mineral in the best form. Since it is a natural food, it can be taken safely in any amount. If you take from four to six tablets a day, however, you won't have much trouble with your teeth.

BREWER'S YEAST

For many years now, nutritionists have prized brewer's yeast as a matchless source of choice protein, natural and organic B vitamins, and minerals.

The cell of brewer's yeast, one of the most minute units of matter in nature, is composed of proteins, carbohydrates, fats, and vitamins and minerals, and resembles in its composition the normal cells of the human body. The yeast cell has within itself, besides all the vitamins of the B-complex, sixteen of the twenty essential amino acids, all eighteen minerals required by the body, and a number of important protein substances—all this in appropriate, health-giving balance, making it one of nature's supreme foods.

In view of the fact that in this country today there is an extensive deficiency in the B-complex vitamins, due partly to the use of devitalized, "nothing" foods, few persons, no matter how physically well they may be, can afford to ignore this very valuable food. It should be made an integral part of the diet, because it is the most concentrated source of nutrition of any known food. It is the very best iron food there is, having more of this vital factor than any other food, not excepting liver. It is specially recommended for those who are anemic or who tire easily.

Brewers' yeast is a superior natural additive to be used in preparing food for the table. If it is added to baked beans, cereals, hamburgers, meat loafs, soups or stews, at the rate of one tablespoon per three servings, it enhances the protein, vitamin, and mineral benefit considerably. Also, it can be mixed with fruit juices, milk, tomato or vegetable juice, or water, and, of course, spread over any other suitable food.

As little as one ounce daily will contribute not only the needful B-complex and vitamins and amino acids, but likewise about 20 percent of the daily protein quantity suggested for an adult. If this amount is included from day to day, a noticeable improvement in well-being should be observed.

LECITHIN

This substance is a union of fat, nitrogen, and phosphorus, and is classified as a phospholipid. It contributes the vitally necessary unsaturated fatty acids commonly known as glycerine and linoleic, linolenic, and phosphoric acids, and the B vitamins choline and inositol. It forms an important part of the tissue in the brain and nerves. In fact, 17 percent of the brain is lecithin.

Lecithin incorporates an emulsifying principle known to have a great ability to break up fats and reduce them to microscopic particles. It is a specific antidote for cholesterol, and maintains it in a state of emulsion. It also insures increased use of vitamins A, D, and E, and helps the body utilize calcium.

Some years ago it was disclosed that cholesterol is one of the causes of hardening of the arteries, and immediately everyone became panicky about cholesterol. Thanks to this unfavorable publicity, we have come to believe that fat in the diet is menacing at best.

It is reported that at present 22 percent of American families are making radical efforts by dietary changes to lower their cholesterol intake—this, notwithstanding the fact that the greater part of the cholesterol content of the body is produced within the body itself, and is required for many bodily activities. It is found in the brain, hair, heart, kidneys, nerves, endocrine glands, skin, and spinal column, as well as the digestive juices.

By eating a high-fat diet, approximately eight hundred milligrams of cholesterol are procured each day. The normal liver, however, will yield about three thousand milligrams per day. So even if you drop foods that contain this substance, the body will keep on producing it.

Besides, living on a low-fat diet may be dangerous, because lecithin plays an important role in the diet, being a part of every body cell and every corpuscle of the blood. Limiting the fats and oils in the diet will lead to a sort of gradual starvation. By all means, curb the carbohydrates, but include the fats and oils.

I should point out here that this product is not a drug, but a granular form of soybean lecithin, free from objectionable elements. It helps relieve stress, and is a 'most important factor for quieting nerves and for general good health. It can induce improved mental poise and a renewed feeling of well-being.

In many cases, when generous amounts of lecithin were added to the diet over an extended period of time, it has been noticed that it benefited the skin by filling it out and softening it and was also effective against other skin problems such as acne, eczema, and psoriasis. It prevented fatigue due to nerve-sheath destruction, promoted greater energy in older people, reduced the cholesterol level in the blood, improved resistance to pneumonia, helped curb nervous exhaustion, and prevented artery and liver impairment. Some people also were better able to withstand virus attacks.

One of the most frequent complaints of men, particularly those past middle age, is nonmalignant enlargement of the prostate gland. More than half of all men past fifty develop this condition, and lecithin has been found very useful in its management. Many investigators have named it a successful remedial treatment.

If sufficient amounts of lecithin are included in the diet, you may be assured that many of the essential raw materials required for the structure and proper functioning of the body cells will be available.

Lecithin is obtainable only in natural foods, not in processed foods. It is present in the natural fats of butter, eggs, and unrefined vegetable oils; or you may get it in a food supplement like lecithin granules, made from soybean oil. This can be added to cereals, fruits, salads, and yogurt, or it can be blended with juices. Seeds—barley seeds, corn seeds, melon seeds, pumpkin seeds, and sunflower seeds—are also good sources.

Other foods high in lecithin are:

beef	safflower oil
corn oil	soybean oil
eggs	wheat germ
nuts	

I regard lecithin as a dietary requisite, and I am confident that, by supplying the necessary materials for cell regeneration, it lengthens human life and makes it more active and vigorous.

SEA KELP

In the ocean is found a plant whose botanical name is *Macrocystis pyrifera,* which is commonly known as kelp. It yields a liberal supply of iodine and is exceedingly fertile in minerals that are imperative for human sustenance. Analyses of kelp indicate that it contains up to twenty-one amino acids, twelve vitamins, and sixty minerals, all naturally balanced.

Why are seaweeds valuable as food? Because in the sea every essential factor necessary for life in its manifold forms is at hand, and there is not and cannot be any nutritional deficit.

Sea plants develop in a mineral-rich environment. According to a Department of the Interior study, "the minor constituents of seaweeds include protein, fat, minerals and vitamins. . . . Seaweeds contain all the mineral elements required for growth." A fractured bone will heal faster when kelp is eaten!

Seaweeds, such as kelp, comprise all the substances found in sea water, which are forthwith passed on to the body, stimulating gland secretion and keeping the blood and tissue fluids from becoming either too acid or too alkaline. It is the ideal mineral supplement.

SUNFLOWER SEEDS

Sunflower seeds head the list of all vegetable concentrates. They are 25 percent protein and are rated in the same class with meat. It is an unusual natural food, about as close to the ideal nutriment as can be obtained from a single source. Nutritionists now generally agree that sunflower seeds are also a good source of vitamins, minerals, calcium, and other food substances.

The oil in these seeds is unsaturated, and by eating them you will obtain the very highest quality of unsaturated fatty acids (vitamin F) that you can consume.

Sunflower seeds are beneficial to eyesight, complexion, fingernails, and act as a curb on high blood pressure and jumpy nerves. Their content of potassium, magnesium and iron is very high. Sunflower seeds are also an important source of vitamin B-complex. . . . The sunflower is in addition a storehouse of vitamins E and D. Sunflower seed.meal proved superior to wheat germ in experiments with animals.[1]

The merit of sunflower seeds is obvious when one examines their vitamin and mineral structure. Nutrients that many people lack are contained in this extraordinary food. Eat some every day. They are of practical use in healing bleeding gums and checking tooth decay, and it is claimed that they even lessen arthritic pains.

YOGURT

I would not do justice to my subject if I failed to say something about that amazing food known as yogurt.

Since biblical times yogurt has been employed primarily as a food, but also to help eliminate putrefaction in the intestinal tract. Nutritional scientists have corroborated this and have shown that yogurt produces lactic acid, which favors the growth of the friendly intestinal bacteria, while inhibiting the development of toxin-producing germs.

It is now thought that yogurt may have powerful anti-cancer properties.

> The harmless, rod-shaped organism which makes yogurt out of milk, Lactobacillus Bulgaricus, turns out to have a potent antitumor activity, according to researchers at the Bulgarian Academy of Sciences in Solla. Injections of LB extracts, they say, can cure several types of experimental cancers, and appear to be effective against human skin tumors.[2]

Yogurt has various advantages over ordinary milk. It is acid in reaction, and this acidity increases with storage.

[1] *Prevention Magazine* (June 1963; April 1963).
[2] Richard D. Townsend, *Let's Talk Health Sense* (Boston: Bruce, Humphries, 1960).

The protein in yogurt is easier to digest and the calcium is more readily assimilated by older folks. It is highly beneficial to persons of all ages. Many mature people who are troubled with immoderate gas find that yogurt is far more helpful than antacids, alkalizers, or bicarbonate of soda, since disturbing bacteria cannot live in the lactic acid of yogurt. This acid is ideal for eliminating toxins and impurities from the body. This may be one of the reasons why constipation is rare in regions where fermented milk foods are used in the basic diet.

It also establishes an acid medium in which most minerals, including calcium and iron, are more completely absorbed. Yogurt manufactures generous amounts of B vitamins in the intestinal tract, which, in turn, keep the entrails vigorous and clean, contribute predigested protein, and facilitate digestion. Yes! Yogurt is a must for those who want to live longer.

Just as surely as two plus two equal four, so the use of the right foods inevitably leads to good health. But, you may ask, how does one begin? With what foods does one start? Quite obviously, one cannot be expected to devise the best possible food regimen on a moment's notice. This will take some time and experience. I do think, however, that readers could speedily put to use a simple guide to foods that will furnish at least the prime factors for glowing health.

Get off to a good start, then, with a high-protein, low-carbohydrate diet rich in meat, fish, and eggs. This is absolutely essential if you want to get the best results. Then add the following supplements daily:

1. One or two tablespoonfuls of brewer's yeast in water, in fruit or vegetable juice, or mixed with other suitable foods. It is a prime source of quality protein, B-complex vitamins, and minerals.

2. One or more tablespoonfuls of unrefined corn oil, for unsaturated fats.

3. One tablespoonful of honey and one of apple cider vinegar in a glass of water. This is principally of benefit to the heart and brain, which operate on glucose, but it also supplies needed acid, vitamins, minerals, and enzymes.

4. Kelp tablets. One five-grain tablet delivers 0.15 milligrams of food iodine, or one and one half times the adult minimum daily requirement. It also provides many trace minerals necessary for health.

Now, if you will make good use of this information, plus a little imagination, you should have no difficulty in planning a wholesome, nutritious diet that will give you a new grip on life.

7

ADULTERATED FOODS AND TOBACCO ARE DANGEROUS

TODAY a great many people are enduring misery from certain serious dietary deficiencies, which cannot be eliminated until nature's way is restored and the present methods of refining foods are abandoned.

Most of the carbohydrate and starchy foods eaten nowadays have been so transformed and contaminated with chemicals that every mouthful consumed includes some traces of harmful substances. The Food and Drug Administration has listed over seven hundred chemicals that are being used in the processing of food, of which only about four hundred are considered safe. There is too much use of what have been termed "empty" or "nothing" foods, foods of little or no value, starchy, artificial, devitalized foods, such as white flour products and white sugar, which are manufactured for profit rather than nourishment.

Practically everything one eats has been bleached, colored, cured, dried, emulsified, enriched, flavored, preserved, refined, stabilized, sweetened, tenderized, or thickened. Only a minimal amount of this food is natural, fresh, or raw.

Linked with these practices is the present-day custom

of harvesting foods before they have fully developed, when their mineral and vitamin content is low. Farmers, too, are more concerned with high crop yields than with nutritional quality; consequently, there has been a steady decline in the amount of nutrients available in food.

Investigators have shown that an analysis of "home-prepared and customer-selected restaurant meals eaten by seventy-one adults in the suburbs of Boston and New York City [indicated] that the intake of niacin came up to only 25 percent of the recommended dietary allowance of the Food and Nutrition Board. Vitamin B-2 intake was only 37 per cent of the recommended amount; vitamin B-1, only 38 per cent; vitamin C, only 52 per cent; calcium, only 63 per cent; and iron, only 72 per cent. These same researchers conducted another sampling of diets across the countryside. Of 3,336 diets analyzed, they were found to be even more deficient in vitamins than those in the New York City and Boston study. In Chicago, a similar study of 7,363 children showed that 72 per cent had unsatisfactory diets."[1]

At the beginning of this section I mentioned that certain carbohydrate and starchy foods were especially detrimental to good health. I would now like to comment on a few of these separately and go into more detail on why and how they affect the body and why you should by all means eliminate them from the diet or use them with extreme moderation.

BREAD

Until whole grains began to be refined, bread was regarded as the "staff of life." Now it has become the most

[1] Linda Clark, *Stay Young Longer* (New York: Devin-Adair Co., 1962).

glaring nutritional absurdity of all. The accumulated testimony against any kind, color, or form of bread is growing more dismaying, day by day. Let's take a closer look at the record.

Bread is substantially a carbohydrate food, and carbohydrate is what puts on excessive weight. It is also an acid food, and contains a substance called phytate that blocks the absorption of calcium. Bread is more fattening than bananas, cream, or potatoes.

A grain of whole wheat contains sixteen minerals: carbon, chlorine, fluorine, hydrogen, iodine, iron, lime, magnesium, manganese, nitrogen, oxygen, phosphorus, potassium, silicon, sodium, and sulphur. The flour millers, however, knock out twelve of these minerals in processing the grains.

Bread manufactured from white, "enriched" flour is void of all life-giving elements, and anyone wishing to build or maintain better health must give up this food for good and all. It contains only three or four of the many B vitamins.

The truth is that the stomachs of many persons are unable to handle bread-starch—and no wonder, when one realizes that our modern "staff of life" contains sodium propionate to kill fungi, chlorine dioxide to bleach it, the jaw-breaking polyoxyethylene-monostearate to prevent staleness and keep it soft and fluffy, plus five or six other chemicals that are added to it at various points during its production.

Various medical writers on food allergies and allergic diseases say that wheat foods are the greatest cause of allergy poisoning and that wheat is the most common food to which patients have shown sensitivity.

Diseases and conditions that can be caused by eating bread and cereal products are: altered liver functions, anemia, cancer, difficult breathing, heart disease, impaired digestion, multiple sclerosis, obesity, polio, rheumatic fever, rheumatoid arthritis.[2]

Other conditions caused in persons allergic to wheat products are abdominal pains, asthma, constipation, diarrhea, eczema, epilepsy, hives, joint pains, migraine headache, and sour stomach.

Diets from which bread and other processed wheat products have been abolished have favorably influenced colitis, sinus trouble, and tuberculosis. If you cut them out, you will feel much better and will catch fewer colds. Too much carbohydrate and starch in the diet can be exceedingly hazardous.

Now—is there a single one of you who is not convinced that you would be far better off giving up bleached white flour, and the products made with it, once and for all?

CITRUS FRUITS

If you will observe people in public eating places, you will note that practically everybody drinks orange or grapefruit juice at breakfast. It has become a national habit—and, I might add, a very questionable habit at that!

When I was a child, the only time you saw an orange was at Christmas, when you usually found one in your Christmas stocking. People did not use very much citrus fruit or drink its juices in those days.

Medical and dental evidence indicates that drinking liberal quantities of citrus fruit juices may injure the teeth

[2] *Prevention* Magazine (December 1962; March 1963; September 1963).

and is sometimes responsible for a runny nose and post-nasal drip. Long-continued daily use of large quantities of citrus fruit or juice can also bring on bleeding gums, fatigue, headaches, loosening of the teeth, and resorption of bone. If your diet happens to be short of B vitamins and minerals, you may likewise develop an increased tendency to pyorrhea.

Moreover, you should at all times use foods that bring about an acid rather than an alkaline urine response. Oranges and grapefruit, or their juices, should be shunned, because the citric acid they contain causes an unwelcome alkaline reaction, and this condition denotes a high blood alkalinity.

I would strongly suggest, however, that if you must use citrus fruits, then eat the whole fruit. We are supposed to eat fruit, not drink it. Canned fruit juices are processed at peak temperatures, which cancels out a great amount of their food benefit. In addition, the coloring material and sugar that they may contain make them undesirable from a health viewpoint.

Citrus fruits may be used in strict moderation as a means of obtaining vitamin C, although a rose-hip product would be a preferable source.

COFFEE

Coffee is one of those substances that, I believe, if taken in moderation, will do you no serious harm, provided you follow a good diet otherwise. All the medical evidence, however, seems to point to the fact that persons who have angina pectoris, arthritis, heart disease, high blood pressure, liver disease, skin problems, or stomach trouble should steer clear of coffee.

The caffeine contained in coffee and tea influences the liver to produce glucose (blood sugar), which, in turn, encourages the pancreas to secrete additional insulin, just as sugar does. However, I don't believe that anyone who drinks one or two cups of coffee a day should necessarily discontinue it. It is the excessive consumption of coffee that puts one in danger.

I once had an experience that demonstrated what an inordinate use of coffee can do. Many years ago, I was in the habit of drinking eight or ten cups of strong coffee daily—and I do mean strong coffee. Eventually I began to suffer from stomach cramps, which occurred every time I ate a meal. By a process of elimination, I discovered that the coffee was doing the mischief. When I gave it up, the pains disappeared. In time, I went back to drinking coffee, but have since limited myself to two or three cups a day, and I have never had a recurrence of the cramps.

There is one big dividend in drinking coffee that may partly make up for its disadvantages. That is, the unusual content of vitamin B in the coffee bean. The information comes from the experiment described in the *Revue Café, Cacao* (October, 1961), performed in the laboratories of the Center for Research in Nutrition of the C. M. R. S. at Bellevue (Seine-et-Vise), France. It was found that coffee is rich in niacin, one of the B fractions, which was originally termed vitamin PP, the PP standing for pellagra preventive.[3]

So it would appear that coffee is not as bad as it is painted.

[3] *Prevention Magazine* (December 1962).

SALT

Salt (sodium) is a mineral that serves to stabilize the acid-base relationship in the body. It is found in all meats, raw fruits, and vegetables, and these foods naturally afford all the food salts we need for health. Meat eaters, especially, can get along very well without additional salt.

Salt also aids the body in its use of potassium, helps to keep calcium in solution, and is required for the utilization of carbohydrates. A lack of salt causes symptoms such as cramps, fatigue, heat stroke, and retarded growth.

> Sodium works with potassium to keep a balance of the acid-base factor in your system; it is needed to maintain a normal balance of water between the cells and fluids. Sodium is also needed to help your nerves respond to stimulation and to help the nerve impulses travel to your muscles. Sodium enables your muscles to contract. Sodium combines with chlorine to improve the health of your blood and lymph. A proper amount of sodium in the blood enables your body to excrete excess carbon dioxide.[4]

However, a great many of today's processed foods are overloaded with salt. Nutritionists say that an excess of salt will cause a retention of fluid in the body and bring about a lack of elasticity of the tissues in the arteries, brain, eyes, heart, muscles, salivary glands, and sex organs. For this reason, many nutrition counselors oppose the use of ordinary table salt.

Because many illnesses are referrable to the use of too much salt, it is customary medical procedure to restrict salt consumption in cases of dropsy, high blood pressure, and heart or kidney diseases, because, since it is an inanimate chemical and not a food, it is treacherous in excess. Salt also contracts the arteries, which prevents an ample

[4] *Health Saver* Magazine (Vol. 5, No. 1, 1962).

flow of blood to the brain, thereby retarding thorough oxygenation.

A low-salt diet has been found beneficial in treatment of deafness, epilepsy, heart conditions, hives, insomnia, migraine headaches, miscarriage, obesity, and sinus trouble. It is supposed to render delivery less difficult in childbirth.

So I urge you to restrict salt or, better still, to exclude it altogether from your diet, especially if you are over fifty. You will obtain plenty of salt in natural foods. By leaving it out in cooking, and not using any at the table, you will discover that you do not miss it after all.

SUGAR

White sugar is 100 percent carbohydrate, and does not contain any protein, vitamins, or minerals. It is the most debased "food" in the American diet. Sugar is an artificial sweet, a powerful, habit-forming stimulant, which cannot possibly build body tissue or improve general health.

Not only is refined white sugar not worth a straw as food, but it is exceedingly injurious to health in the volume in which many people consume it. In 1900, the average consumption of sugar in the United States per person per year was about nine pounds. Now it is about 150 pounds. Think of it! This is sixty to seventy-five pounds more sugar than is required for ideal energy and subsistence.

A great quantity of this surplus sugar is derived from bakery products, jams and jellies, candy, and soft drinks (of which the American people are the largest consumers in the world). These sugar-saturated, carbonated beverages, which also contain caffeine, are taken by adults, teenagers, and even children. The injurious substances that they contain eat away at the body's accessible reserves of nerve-calming B-complex vitamins. Soft drinks also damage teeth and digestive membrane.

Most of these products "are full of artificial flavorings, colorings, and preservatives. As much as ninety percent of some candy is a concoction of preservatives, anti-oxidents, stabilizers, thickeners, buffers, acids, synthetic coloring, flavoring, and other chemical agents.[5]

When sugar is consumed, the blood-sugar level rises very rapidly; soon after, however, the blood sugar drops far below normal limits, due to oversecretion of insulin by the pancreas. This condition is known as hypoglycemia, or low blood sugar, and it has become a menace to the national health. It is even more prevalent than its opposite—diabetes. Hypoglycemia is called the "hunger disease," because, when too much sugar or starch is used, it induces an abnormal desire for food, which is accompanied by fatigue in many cases.

The numerous recorded symptoms of this disorder are: alcoholism, allergies, anxiety, arthritis, asthma, crying spells, depression, fatigue, heart palpitation, hunger, migraine headache, nervousness, peptic ulcer, rheumatic fever, and feelings of weakness. Hypoglycemia also simulates the symptomatic appearance of many other diseases.

Excessive intake of beverages containing caffeine is a common cause of this condition. Statistics indicate that low blood sugar is one of the characteristics of schizophrenia, and it should be noted that a definite mutual relationship has been shown to exist between low blood sugar and certain other types of mental illness. Anyone suffering from this disease must give up alcohol, candy, coffee, ice cream, macaroni, noodles, pies, puddings, soft drinks, sugar, and syrup.

As far back as the glacial age, man has been plagued by

---

[5] Richard D. Townsend, *Let's Talk Health Sense* (Boston: Bruce, Humphries, 1960).

cavities in the teeth. Today, in the United States—a high-incidence country—more than nine out of every ten persons, including over 90 percent of all school-age children, have some dental caries; and it is estimated that, at any one time, at least seven hundred million unfilled cavities await the dentist's drill.

Leading dentists agree that the most destructive decay agents in the mouth are the bacteria that thrive on refined white sugar, creating acids that are chiefly responsible for tooth decay. The disease bacteria must have food in order to flourish, and the foods they go for in particular are carbohydrates, especially sugars.

To prevent tooth decay, it is necessary to arrest the harmful process at some point, and scientists have put forward many theories on how best to accomplish this. However, scientists and nutritionists are in agreement that dental caries are caused by unsound nutrition.

It appears that vitamins A and C are required for the formation of enamel on the teeth. Calcium and phosphorus are necessary for rebuilding body tissues and especially for good tooth structure. Finally, the B-complex vitamins are very important in that they check decay and guard mouth health. Refined white sugar not only disturbs the calcium-phosphorus balance in the body but displaces or dilutes these important vitamins and other nutrients.

> Thus, the more sugar consumed, the less opportunity for getting essential nutrients into the diet. If sugar is furnished as a replacement of proteins, fats, minerals and vitamins, then serious physiological consequences follow.[6]

Some writers on nutrition claim that refined and processed foods that are overloaded with sugar are directly

[6] E. M. Abrahamson and A. W. Pezet, *Body, Mind and Sugar* (New York: Holt, Rinehart & Winston, 1951).

connected with poliomyelitis. Polio epidemics have occurred throughout the world in recent years only in those
regions where excessive amounts of sugar are used, and
are unheard of in lands with insignificant sugar consumption.

It has also been shown that a close relationship exists
between this serious disease and deficiency of the B-complex vitamins, and it is well known that sugar destroys
the B vitamins in the intestinal tract. This means that,
if you use white sugar, you are bound to have such a
deficiency, because the body must draw them from other
sources in order to assimilate the sugar.

Sugar, white flour, and refined and processed foods in
general, by undermining the heart and the vasomotor
nerves that regulate the tension in the blood vessels, may
thus be an important factor in causing hardening of the
arteries and heart disease.

Finally, as far back as 1929, Dr. F. G. Banting, the
discoverer of insulin, noted that the incidence of diabetes
in the United States was increasing proportionately with
the per capita consumption of cane sugar.

The prohibitions against sugar may be set aside, however, when natural sugars are used. The best form is the
natural sugar found in dates, figs, and other fruits, honey,
and blackstrap molasses, since these foods contain the
thiamine (vitamin B-1) that is needed to help the body
metabolize the sugar.[7] Substituting natural carbohydrates
for white sugar and starch will benefit anyone's health.
As with all sweets, moderation is indicated.

---

[7] Health food shops also have available a light-colored sugar
under the trade name Turbinado Sugar, also called "raw" sugar.
Since this product has not been treated with the many chemicals
to which highly processed sugar is exposed, it still contains many
minerals and other nutrients found in sugar cane. Used sparingly,
it makes a relatively safe, delicious substitute for refined sugar.

TOBACCO

At this point, I would like to digress for a few moments to write something on the subject of tobacco. Having used it for many years, I believe that I can speak with some authority as to its effects on the human system.

For a great many years, I had suffered from a chronic cough. Although I suspected that tobacco was the cause, I didn't want to give it up, and I was reluctant to admit this, even to myself. I had received medical treatment for the cough from time to time, without appreciable results.

Finally, I was compelled to face the fact that my health was being seriously undermined. I quit "the weed" seven years ago, because I simply got tired of feeling bad. A few weeks later, the cough cleared up, and it has never returned. Another result that I noticed was that my breathing improved within two or three months after stopping smoking.

Tobacco is a habit-forming substance and is one of the most deadly poisons known to man. Smoking is self-induced air pollution and presents a hazard to health, even to life itself. This has been found to be the case by every responsible medical and health organization that has investigated the subject in the United States and abroad. Evidence now reveals that tobacco smoking has such a thoroughly harmful effect on health that it should be abolished. If you smoke a pack of cigarettes a day, you inhale about four hundred milligrams of nicotine a week, which, if taken in a single injection, would kill you immediately.

In cigarette smoking, one of the chief causes of local irritation of the throat, aside from the tobacco itself, is the chemical acrelin impregnated in the paper. A survey indicated that cigarette smokers have 167 percent higher incidence of nose and throat irritations, a 300 percent greater ratio of coughs, and 65 percent more colds.

Everything in the nutritional literature indicates that tobacco is especially detrimental to the adrenal glands and destroys vitamin C in the body. Smoking weakens masculine virility and is one of the causes of prostatic hypertrophy (enlarged prostate gland).

The nervous system is influenced injuriously by heavy smoking. Stomach disorders; skin ailments; damage to teeth and gums; impairment of the senses of hearing, eyesight, smell, and taste; shortness of breath; muscular fatigue; delayed reflexes; and adverse effects on kidneys and blood sugar are a few more of the likely physical consequences of smoking. Symptoms of low blood sugar have been completely relieved when tobacco was discontinued.

Tobacco smoking is also a prime cause of difficulty in blood circulation, especially in the lower limbs, as it narrows the blood vessels. Cardiovascular diseases common during and after middle age have been diagnosed as resulting from habitual smoking.

> Of interest to expectant mothers should be the following: In an article in the New York *Mirror* (July 16, 1962), the Public Health Service said that "prematurity, stillbirths, and brain damage have been linked with smoking, [as well as] some previously unsuspected events of pregnancy and delivery." Dr. Richard L. Masland, Director of the National Institute of Neurological Diseases and Blindness, stated that "infants weighing 5½ pounds or less were considered to be premature, and ... the early findings in regard to effects of smoking by mothers showed birthweight was inversely proportional to the reported amount of smoking."[8]

[8] *Health Bulletin* (June 15, 1963).

Despite the fact that the vested interests in tobacco are injecting confusion into the discussion, clear indications that cancer of the larynx and the lungs is closely associated with cigarette smoking can no longer be seriously questioned. The grim fact is that, in 1966, forty-two thousand men and eight thousand women were killed by lung cancer. Today only 5 percent of lung cancer victims are saved.

There can be no doubt that smoking is one of the toughest habits to break, so if you have made unsuccessful attempts to stop it (and what smoker hasn't?), very likely it is not that you lack the will power to accomplish your purpose, but that your interest in giving it up has not been sufficiently aroused. Mere resolution is not enough. You must first be convinced, as I was, of the dire threat to your health posed by tobacco, and then your will power will do the job.

I began by quitting for one month at a time, and renewing my resolve each month for five or six months. By that time I had it licked. Truthfully, I was agreeably surprised how easy it was. If I were you, I would drop smoking—but quick!

8

CLEAN—INSIDE AND OUT

AS my knowledge of what foods to eat or avoid gradually increased, it became clear to me that no program for health, no matter how elaborate, would be adequate unless one adopted some efficient method of keeping the inside of the body just as clean as the outside. I can think of nothing more important to your well-being.

The late Dr. Alexis S. Carrel, renowned biologist and the world's greatest authority on cell hygiene, gave profound study to this subject. In his book *Man the Unknown,* he demonstrated that vigor and vitality will continue indefinitely as long as thorough hygiene is practiced and appropriate foods are supplied daily. If they receive the essential nutrition they need, and if all poisons are removed from them without delay, tissue cells can be kept alive indefinitely, Dr. Carrel stated.

This subject is not extensively treated in books and articles on diet and nutrition, on the assumption, perhaps, that if one eats a good diet, thorough elimination will most likely follow. Nonetheless, it is my considered opinion that in these times, when even the best foods are loaded with additives and chemicals, some of which may be cancer-causing, a regular flushing out of the internal organs is not only advisable but imperative.

Theoretically, all disease has its origin in an impure bloodstream. Biliousness, bladder and kidney disturbances, infections, bronchitis, colds, influenza, constipation, indigestion, headaches, liver disorders, and rheumatism are some of the more familiar manifestations that warn of an intestinal tract that is congested and overburdened with a mass of irritating and deadly waste products.

These conditions are mainly caused by excessive use of concentrated starch, such as white bread, pastries, and spaghetti; and other refined carbohydrates, such as white sugar. Alcohol, coffee, tea, and carbonated beverages should also be taken in extreme moderation, because all such foodstuffs encourage the accumulation of a vast multitude of disease bacteria in the bowel, which should not be there and which, in turn, produce a lazy bowel, overburdened kidneys, and toxic agitation in the stomach and digestive tract. When normal activities of the stomach and intestines are interfered with, poisons are detained in the body, which can result in a state of autointoxication.

The body has four main channels of elimination—the bowels, the kidneys, the lungs, and the pores of the skin. Maintaining these outlets active is highly important, simply because any bodily function operates better when it is kept clean. It is just as important for health as eating a balanced diet.

Cleansing the body is not complicated, but it will require, for most people, a change in certain dietary details. A person who eats properly and moderately, who maintains clean, healthy bowels, whose elimination and metabolism indicate smooth functioning of the internal organs, will have gone a long way toward preventing cancer, or colds, or any other disease, for that matter.

Constipation is one of the causes of premature old age. It is a sign of dehydration. The human body is approximately 60 percent water, by weight, and the full-grown body loses about three quarts of water daily. Many middle-aged and older people are dehydrated, which is some-times indicated by dry, withered skin. Lack of water at the proper time may be responsible for this condition.

Water enters into the formation of every tissue, and is one of our major foods. It is best taken while the stomach is empty. An average person may require six to ten glasses of liquid daily, part of which can be obtained from certain substantial, mineral-rich, unrefined foods, such as apples, cantaloupe, fresh fruits, honeydew melon, vegetable juices, and watermelon, as well as pure water. Restrict liquids at meals, however, because food is digested by gastric juices, not by water.

Along with the foods just mentioned, the B-complex vitamins are urgently needed for healthy functioning of the bowels. These vitamins are necessary for a clean, healthy intestinal tract with a normal production of energy. Similarly, protein is essential to strengthen the intestinal muscles. If these muscles are undernourished, they may become flabby and will be unable to contract and expand as they should.

The chief cause of persistent constipation in our so-ciety is the widespread addiction to laxatives.

Millions of us have become laxative addicts. The American people spent 162 million dollars for laxatives last year (1961). Indiscriminate use of laxatives is foolish, sometimes dangerous. They interfere with the proper absorption of foods from the small intestine, and with the reabsorption of critically important sodium and potassium in the large intestine. . . . All laxatives depress production of the B vitamins in the large intes-tine. Moreover, many widely-used laxatives are power-ful irritants. When laxatives push foods through the large intestine too quickly, precious potassium is lost. If the loss is severe, breathing muscles and heart may be hit.[1]

Fortunately, however, in addition to proper diet, there is a very effective cleansing procedure which you can follow very easily yourself. It is nothing more than a natural, internal bath, which is dependable and entirely automatic in its cleansing action. It need not be used very frequently; perhaps four to six times a year will suffice. If you try it, I think you will agree that it is unsurpassed. It is a wonderful cleanser, absolutely harmless, does not cause the slightest distress, and I can personally testify to its effectiveness. Here it is:

Add two level teaspoons of common table salt to a measured quart (32 ounces) of warm water. Water and salt must be exactly measured. Water should be warm, not hot. Drink the solution on an empty stomach a half hour before breakfast. Drink the entire quart, a glassful at a time, within the space of four or five minutes if possible. Lying on your right side for about a quarter of an hour will encourage the solution to pass along the intestinal tract. In about one hour, or less, the entire quart of salt water (together with considerable waste) should be eliminated.[2]

As you acquire the good habit of eating only basically protective foods, nature will eventually correct any abnormal condition and restore the regular, normal action of the intestinal tract.

[1] *Reader's Digest* (November 1962).
[2] John X. Loughran, *90 Days to a Better Heart* (New York: Devin-Adair Co.. 1958).

9

YOU CAN HAVE ATTRACTIVE SKIN

THE skin, like all other parts of the body, is formed of protein. Naturally, therefore, a diet ample in protein is essential to keep the skin healthfully in bloom.

It is very important to keep the skin clean, both externally and internally, to prevent the accumulation of toxic wastes in the pores. Therefore, the first step in achieving a fine skin should be treatment from within by consuming an adequate amount of the best protein foods (meat, fish, and eggs), which replenish all the essential amino acids necessary to keep skin healthy.

A good supply of eggs, muscle and organ meats, and seafood in the diet, supplemented daily by a tablespoon or more of cod liver oil, corn oil, olive oil, safflower oil, or wheat germ oil, to provide vital unsaturated fatty acids, makes a superior internal food bonus to attractive skin. Linoleic acid, a constituent of corn oil, has been shown to be beneficial to eczema. Even psoriasis has been favorably affected by the addition of salad oils to the diet. In fact, beautiful skin and superb health are impossible without appropriate fats.

Studies by leading dermatologists reveal that the B

vitamins thiamine (B-1), riboflavin (B-2), and pyridoxine (B-6), are especially important to skin health. It appears that the body needs substantial quantities of the
B vitamins regularly to provide the skin with an adequate
defense against many types of dermatoses (skin diseases).
To reinforce your regular diet, a daily supplement of
brewer's yeast is your best source of properly balanced
B vitamins. Minerals are also required to keep the skin
glowing and alive-looking, so use apricots, blackstrap
molasses, leafy greens, and sunflower seeds, as well as
kelp tablets for natural iodine and all organic trace minerals. It can make the difference between a jaded look
and a youthful one.

Special attention should be paid to foods that sustain
steady blood circulation, such as those containing vitamin
A, vitamin B-complex, vitamin C, and the minerals calcium, iodine, and iron, because the skin tone hinges on
circulation.

Exclude from your food intake all sweets, candies,
pastries, and soft drinks, because refined sugar is very
harmful to skin health, due to the fact that it encourages
the growth of bacteria. Use honey for sweetening. Salt,
too, is detrimental to skin beauty because of its drying
effect, causing wrinkles. Banish white flour products, such
as bread, cake, crackers, and doughnuts, and avoid fried
foods. Try to keep in mind that what you eat has a decisive effect on your skin, as well as on your general health
and happiness.

In your efforts to take care of or improve your skin,
the harm commercial deodorants and cosmetics can do
should not be overlooked. You risk the health of your
skin by using these products because the detergents, lubri-
cants, and perfume they are composed of can cause skin
irritation, blisters, rashes, and other skin conditions. It

is further reported that bleaching, cleansing, and freckle creams frequently cause the most disagreeable skin reactions. Play safe! Your local health food shop can supply natural, safe deodorants and cosmetics which are free of irritating chemical additives.

10

EXERCISE CHECKS PREMATURE AGING

WHILE eating wholesome food is obviously essential for maintaining a good physical condition, it is also true that the best food imaginable cannot be efficiently absorbed into the system without some form of exercise. Mild exercise also adds to the benefits derived from vitamin-mineral supplements by aiding in their digestion.

Generally speaking, you do not require strenuous or laborious exercise for good health, although body functions must be disciplined if their power is to be sustained. A reasonable amount of moderate physical exertion is important to health and is especially necessary for those who are incapable, for serious reasons, of controlling or arranging an appropriate diet. If you would have the joy of feeling good, then, you must not neglect this most important activity.

The major job that exercise performs is to oxygenate the body. Another good result of exercise is that it quickens blood circulation, dilates the arteries and veins of the heart, and serves to keep the arteries supple, thus guarding against arteriosclerosis and other symptoms of advancing age. It is a known fact that people who exercise regularly are much less prone to heart attacks.

Exercise also improves the posture by maintaining good muscular firmness throughout the body, especially in the legs. To some extent, too, exercise of the muscles will help strengthen the nerves. If practised regularly, it will do a great deal to relax them and bring about inner calm. Other desirable effects of habitual exercise are improvement of bowel action, relief of fatigue and tension, aid in taking off excess weight, inducing sound sleep, reduction of the cholesterol level, and lowering the pulse, which helps to protect against strokes.

Recently, scientists have proved by experiments with animals that the stabilizing effects of exercise may retard or even interrupt the growth of cancer. Exercise is very beneficial to body cells, rendering them less vulnerable to destructive influences that can cause and sustain cancer.

I recommend walking and dancing as ideal forms of regular, pleasant exercise, which meet practically all bodily requirements. Either of these physical activities uses most of the vital muscles, and both are so mild that anyone can enjoy them. Dancing is thought to be even better than walking, because it is performed to music and thus is rhythmical.

According to Dr. William Brady, writing in the Chicago *Daily News* (January 2, 1958), a brisk walk of several miles encourages the body to store up calcium. It also enhances the absorption of vitamin A and the secretion of digestive juices, enzymes, and hormones, and it stimulates other bodily functions. There is not a single part of the body that is not greatly aided and strengthened by muscular effort, and exercise is therefore one of the best remedies for an ailing body. Muscles that are exercised every day age more slowly. If possible, walk for a minimum of thirty minutes, or even as far as two miles, each day.

The object of walking is to relax the mind. You should therefore not permit yourself even to think while you walk; but divert yourself by the objects surrounding you. . . . Habituate yourself to walk very far. The Europeans value themselves on having subdued the horse to the uses of man; but I doubt whether we have not lost more than we have gained, by the use of this animal. No one has occasioned so much the degeneracy of the human body. An Indian goes on foot near as far in a day, for a long journey, as an enfeebled white does on his horse; and he will tire the best horses. There isno habit you will value so much as that of walking far without fatigue.

That was written by Thomas Jefferson, back in 1785.

One need not spend hours in daily calisthenics. The ordinary movements required in carrying out normal tasks, such as bathing or showering, doing housework, and getting dressed, with a one- or two-mile walk worked in, should ordinarily suffice to keep one fit. However, in view of the fact that suppleness of the spine has a significant influence on the nervous energy supplied to most of the muscles and organs of the body, I wish to suggest that you try one of the best and simplest exercises there is: Hang by your arms from a bar, with the full weight suspended, for from six to ten seconds. This extends the spinal column slightly and has the effect of drawing the body out to its full length. By doing this, you can avoid chronic fatigue and gain many other health benefits.

I recommended this exercise to a lady who had sustained a severe back injury in an automobile accident. About a month later, she wrote me a letter, which I quote in part as follows:

Now I have some news—very good for me, and I know that you likewise will be pleased to hear of it. The exercise you recommended—hanging by the arms in order to stretch the spine from top to bottom—is actually doing wonders! . . . What an amazing difference it made in the weight-bearing areas of my back!

All along I have felt that what I really needed was stretching, manipulation, etc., instead of diathermy treatments and injections. I had moments when the pressure was almost too much to bear, and the injections [gave] only a temporary relief. And now, . . . [with] this very simple exercise, for the first time in many months I have considerably less pain. To say nothing of the favourable psychological effect it is having on me. . . . It's incredible that the simple exercise you recommended should work wonders!

To supplement the exercise described above, here are a few more easy but effective exercises, each of which takes only a few seconds.

FOR ARM MUSCLES:
Press one clenched fist forcibly into the other palm.

FOR STOMACH MUSCLES:
Pull in the stomach, and suck the diaphragm up until the whole diaphragm is flat. Release little by little. Do it gently the first few times to avoid possible lightheadedness. Many movie stars do this exercise to improve posture and flatten the tummy.

FOR MUSCLE TONE:
After a bath or shower, loop the towel behind your neck. Then pull your chin in, pull forward on both ends of the towel and resist with your neck, as hard as you can, just six seconds. Do it only once. Now slide the towel down to the small of your back. While pulling forward on the towel, resist by contracting the muscles in your buttocks and belly. Loop the towel under your toes and pull up with both hands while your toes push down. Hold it for six seconds, then let go. Once on each foot and you're done for the day.*

* Linda Clark, *Stay Young Longer* (New York: Devin-Adair Co., 1962).

A slant board, a device that raises the feet twelve or fifteen inches higher than the head, will increase blood circulation to the face and head, by counteracting the force of gravity.

For those who prefer more active or strenuous exercise, nothing excels weight lifting. As a beginning, you can use a barbell without additional weights. The bar itself weighs about fifteen or twenty pounds. You can gradually increase the weight as your ability indicates.

The exercise consists in standing with feet apart, then squatting. Grasp the bar with the palms toward the body. Then stand, while at the same time lifting the bar to the chest, then above the head, then lowering it to the chest, and to the floor. Do eight to twelve repetitions once a day. This activates all the muscles, and you should notice an increase in strength very soon.

11

MORE REST—LESS TENSION

ONE hears and reads a great deal about the beneficial effects of exercise for physical fitness. What I believe to be equally as important is the necessity for rest and relaxation, especially for those who are overwrought or in poor health.

Do you frequently get up in the morning so tired that you feel as though you had been pulled through a keyhole, and not knowing how you can make it through the day? If so, the first question to ask yourself is how much sleep you are getting each night, because fatigue can be a symptom of organic disease. It is the most common complaint that doctors hear.

Rest and sleep are as important as exercise, food, and pure air. You cannot expect your body to maintain its energy and endurance on little sleep, because it must have proper rest to relieve weariness and revitalize the tissues. Also, the more rested the body, the better the blood circulation.

Loss of sleep is in fact very injurious to health and accelerates aging. People who sleep five or six hours a night, and appear to evade the consequences, often find themselves in impaired health later on. The statistical standard in the United States is from six to nine hours of sleep a night. Most people need at least eight hours' sleep, and some require more. Personal experience over many years has taught me that from ten to twelve hours of rest, not necessarily taken all at one time, make me feel my best. As Cervantes said in *Don Quixote,* "Now blessings light on him that first invented sleep! It covers a man all over, thoughts and all, like a cloak; 'tis meat for the hungry, drink for the thirsty, heat for the cold, and cold for the hot, and the balance that sets the king and the shepherd, the fool and the wise man even."

It is true that recreation is essential for good health, and that food can offset loss of sleep to some degree, but there is nothing that can actually substitute for sufficient relaxation. Requirements may vary with different individuals, but if one does not get the amount of rest he needs, his life expectancy will definitely be decreased. Lost sleep can never be regained.

For good, relaxed sleep, calcium (a nerve soother), vitamin B-complex, vitamin C, and lactic acid (from milk products) are helpful. In general, the more hours devoted to sleep prior to midnight, the better rested you will be.

In addition to a first-rate diet, the secret of sustained, buoyant health of body and mind during the later years of life is to provide for a healthy balance between exercise and rest. In these later years especially, it is wise to permit oneself short intervals of complete relaxation. Best of all, a regular daily nap is a wonderful youth conserver and can add up to ten years to the life span.

12

CORONARY DISEASE—LEADING KILLER

AS one grows older, the body uses less oxygen, and consequently there is a tendency for poisons to accumulate, especially in the intestinal tract. These poisons ravage the body, hardening the arteries, inhibiting breathing and blood circulation, and causing other characteristics of old age. The mental stress and anxiety brought about by these conditions places an additional strain on the unprotected cardiovascular system.

Pneumonia was formerly the greatest cause of death among older people, but nowadays coronary artery disease is the top killer of persons over the age of fifty. Over 17 million Americans are affected to some degree, and more than half of all deaths in this country can be traced to this malady. In addition, 40 percent of all persons seventy-five or over are troubled with high blood pressure, a condition brought about by narrowing of the arterial walls.

There are many determining circumstances that contribute to the development of arteriosclerosis (hardening of the arteries), and it appears that no one particular factor can be charged with the blame. Among foods, however, white flour products are regarded as substances that specifically encourage this disease.

Arteriosclerosis can result from an abnormal thickening and hardening of the arterial walls due to calcium precipitation, which generally occurs in the later years of life. Another contributory factor is believed to be cholesterol, a constituent of animal fat, which produces a solid, waxlike substance that adheres to the walls of the arteries. And yet, as we have mentioned earlier, the Eskimos living at the Arctic Circle, who eat extraordinary amounts of animal fat, are widely known to be exempt from arteriosclerosis and heart conditions.

Another form of this disease is cerebral arteriosclerosis, an inelasticity of the blood vessels in the brain, which ultimately brings about mental decline, lapse of memory, and sometimes paralysis. It is of rather frequent occurrence.

If you suffer from hardening of the arteries, a diet including fat meat *without salt,* baked or boiled potatoes with butter, and fresh fruit will help to rebuild them. In addition, moderate exercise in the open air will bring back elasticity to the arteries, at least to some degree. Remember, poor circulation constantly puts additional stress on the heart.

Then, too, an insufficient supply of the B vitamins biotin, choline, and inositol appears to be a significant factor in the onset of this malady. Investigation has shown that many cases of hardened arteries are being successfully treated with these vitamins. Further improvement is obtained by adding daily three hundred to five hundred milligrams of vitamin C, with the bioflavonoids, which help to oxygenate the heart. When these vitamins are generously combined with the proper diet, arteriosclerosis may be gradually corrected.

Serious heart conditions, such as coronary occlusion and coronary thrombosis, as well as impaired circulation and stroke, can result from atherosclerosis (thickening of the arteries), a type of arteriosclerosis generally attributed to an accumulation of excess cholesterol in these blood vessels. However, it has never been proved that such deposits of cholesterol actually bring about this disorder. In fact, a study made at the Johns Hopkins University School of Medicine indicated that cholesterol is not the primary cause.[1]

Sunflower seeds and sunflower seed oil are extensively used in some of the European countries, notably Russia. Tests made on a considerable number of people in those countries indicated that sunflower seed oil was exceptionally beneficial in cases of atherosclerosis and heart disease. All were given proteins, carbohydrates, and vitamins, plus sunflower seed oil. It was reported that after the oil was used for thirty days, there was a marked improvement in the chemistry of the blood and a lower cholesterol count. Heart symptoms also abated and were noticed less often. Improved bowel activity was also recorded.

Atherosclerosis is the most prevalent form of cardiovascular disease in the United States, and 25 percent of all deaths in this country are now attributed to it. Healthy persons well along in years may escape atherosclerosis by the regular use of natural vitamin C, lecithin, salad oils, and wheat germ in goodly quantities.

One of the more prevalent forms of cardiovascular disorder, caused by impaired blood circulation, is varicose veins. This disease is especially common in persons past middle age. Oddly, however, this very distressing and painful degenerative disorder is becoming much more frequent among young people. The veins most often affected are the ones closest to the skin, which receive a limited degree of support from the muscles and bones.

This is one ailment, however, that you can prevent by giving up certain injurious habits that you may now have.

[1] Reported in the Baltimore *Evening Sun*, February 28, 1963.

For example, one of the more detrimental things you can do for the good health of the veins is to stand in one spot for long periods, as when ironing, washing dishes, or cooking. Whenever possible, sit down while you work, or else you will be inviting the possibility of varicose veins.

Another practice that leads to varicose veins is wearing tight garters, corsets, or girdles. These slow down blood circulation, even if they are not irksome. Crossing your legs does the same thing. Varicose veins can develop into more serious complications if disregarded.

After every possible effort has been made to eliminate whatever has contributed to the onset of varicose veins— long hours of standing, insufficient exercise, and tight clothing—an examination of your diet is in order. Since the food you take into your body will largely determine the health of the veins and arteries, a high-protein, low-carbohydrate diet is indicated. In addition, supplements of the following concentrated nutrients are suggested:

VITAMIN A
This vitamin is extremely valuable for the health of the linings of all body organs.

VITAMIN C
This substance is absolutely necessary for the durability of blood-vessel walls. A deficiency of vitamin C, not critical enough to cause bleeding, can bring on deterioration of the veins, which give way and twist into various distorted shapes visible on the surface of the skin.

VITAMIN P (THE BIOFLAVONOIDS)
This nutrient is associated with vitamin C and always occurs with it in natural foods. Since it provides effective protection against varicosed conditions, be sure to use a vitamin C product that incorporates the bioflavonoids.

VITAMIN E
Another substance that is essential for the health of the blood vessels, vitamin E has been used successfully in the treat-

ment of varicose veins, as it prevents blood clots from forming. It also opens up areas of venous obstruction and reduces the strain on overworked veins. It helps shrink the swollen veins to normal size, thus relieving congestion and pain. Its curative power is second to none.

High blood pressure is implicated in three fourths of the deaths resulting from heart and kidney disease that occur annually in the United States, and it is becoming an increasingly important health problem in its own right.

Too much salt is believed to have a definite negative influence on blood pressure and the condition of the arteries, because salt encourages an abnormal accumulation of fluids in the body. The most reasonable course for those troubled with high blood pressure, it seems, would be for them to limit their salt intake—or, better still, to give up salt and very salty foods entirely. There is enough natural salt already present in food to satisfy the body's needs.

Another method of coping with high blood pressure is to step up the amount of acid taken daily through the use of apple cider vinegar or ascorbic acid (vitamin C), cranberries, or grapes, or their juices. Garlic, which is a blood purifier, has also been used successfully in treating this disorder; it is available in capsule form. Additional calcium should also be taken to help maintain relaxation.

On the other hand, I think that many people worry too much about their blood pressure, thus causing themselves needless anxiety and unhappiness.

When one reflects upon the universal refinement of popular foods, it is not surprising that the number of people afflicted with arteriosclerosis, cancer, diabetes, heart disease, and high blood pressure has risen so alarmingly since the time when grains were first processed, and vitamin E and all the B-complex vitamins began to be thrown out in the process. If not with reference to these practices, how can one explain the extraordinary increase in these degenerative diseases?

Nature replenishes all the cells of the body as they wear out (with a few exceptions, such as the cells of the heart and brain, which must last a lifetime); and, unless interrupted by disease or injury, this cell activity should continue indefinitely. Owing to some elusive factor, however, the replacement procedure is hampered, and the body begins to age. This phenomenon is now being thoroughly studied, and it is possible that the aging process may eventually be controlled. Therefore, it is more important than ever that the untimely heart attacks that have begun to strike down young and middle-aged people be prevented. To do this, however, a rearrangement of food habits will be necessary for most people, as well as more careful attention to their mode of living.

Degenerative disorders are five times as prevalent today as they were seventy years ago. In the United States, in the era prior to 1920, coronary heart disease was uncommon in people over fifty, and until 1896 it was practically unknown. Today heart disease affects about five million people and takes over a half million lives annually in America—that is, nearly fourteen hundred deaths every twenty-four hours! According to Adelle Davis, a leading nutritionist, this disease, which is caused by faulty eating, "is responsible for more invalids than any other sickness."[2] As a result of the increased incidence of this malady, Americans sixty years of age or over now have a life expectancy lower than that of a hundred years ago.

[2] Adelle Davis, *Let's Eat Right to Keep Fit* (New York: Harcourt, Brace & World, 1954).

Heart disease deals a death blow to one man in five among those over fifty.

The heart is one of the most resilient and powerful organs of the body. For this reason, there is a great deal of debate as to the cause of the widespread heart degeneration among our people. Some authorities hold that cholesterol, which clings to arterial walls and hinders the flow of blood to the heart, is the principal cause. Others dispute this theory, because there are still many vexing problems in connection with this matter.

The fact is that cholesterol is of the highest significance to the body, in that it actually preserves the arteries. Cholesterol is also an essential part of certain specific tissues, such as those of the kidney, liver, and nerves. Consequently, there is serious doubt concerning the entire theory that fat in the diet causes heart disease. Moreover, there is no convincing scientific evidence to establish as a certainty that eating fat brings about obstruction of the arteries. Actually, fat is indispensable for good nutrition because it supplies a concentrated source of energy. Further, some fats contribute the essential vitamins A and D, as well as highly important fatty acids.

Dr. Benjamin P. Sandler, a well-known physician who specializes in this field, contends that starch and carbohydrates tend to lower blood-sugar levels, and this in turn gives rise to heart disease and polio. He does not believe that fat in the diet causes arteriosclerosis, which is assumed to be responsible for the recent rise in heart disease. The low-carbohydrate diet he devised has been effective in many cases in relieving heart pain and in warding off its recurrence.[3]

Other authorities agree that sugar is more closely related

[3] Benjamin P. Sandler, *How to Prevent Heart Attacks* (Milwaukee: Lee Foundation for Nutritional Research, 1958).

to the incidence of heart attacks than is fat. It is believed that refined sugar causes an inordinate quantity of fat molecules to be deposited in the bloodstream.

It has been found that a deficiency of vitamin E also has a great deal to do with bringing on heart distress. In recent years, Dr. E. V. Shute and his associates in London, Ontario, Canada, have conclusively demonstrated that thousands of patients with all types of heart ailments— angina pectoris, coronary occlusion, coronary thrombosis, heart injury caused by rheumatic fever, and other variations—repeatedly made striking improvement when vitamin E was included in the diet. In many cases of angina pectoris, pain was eliminated and patients were able to return to profitable activity. Building a better heart also yields an unexpected bonus of serenity and well-being difficult to express in words.

The heart pumps several tons of blood every day, and practically no type of physical exertion can overtax a healthy heart, let alone injure it. But to have a strong heart and excellent blood, one must have a sound digestive system and eat the best possible food. If you wish to avoid heart and circulatory ailments, put yourself on a high-protein, low-carbohydrate diet for life.

Meat, fish, and eggs were once considered objectionable in heart cases involving high blood pressure. Today, however, these foods are recognized as high-class proteins, which are both desirable and appropriate for inclusion in the diet.

Here are some additional suggestions:

Take daily as a food supplement, preferably at breakfast, 2 to 4 tablespoons of lecithin granules. Add B complex in its potent form to your diet—brewer's yeast. Add daily 25,000 units of vitamin A and 150 milligrams of vitamin

C. Take 2 tablespoons of soy, corn, or safflower oil daily. Include 2 to 4 tablespoons of wheat germ.[4]

Finally, make use of kelp, which provides that all-important food, iodine, and other mineral factors so essential to good heart tone.

[4] Linda Clark, *Stay Young Longer* (New York: Devin-Adair Co., 1962).

13

RESPIRATORY DISEASES CAN DAMAGE HEART AND LUNGS

ALTHOUGH it has troubled man for centuries, asthma is still scarcely understood, and no practical means of curing it has been formulated. It is primarily a lingering disease, which is usually caused by some allergy. Asthma is characterized by difficulty in breathing due to contraction of the air passages, which is brought on by spasms of the diaphragm. It can be influenced by inner conflicts or tensions and by nervous disorders.

About half the cases reported are caused by dust inhalation or by the ingestion of drugs and certain foods. Very seldom is the root cause known, but, as in any allergy, there is an unnatural reaction to normally harmless substances, such as eggs, milk, and wheat.

The failure to use the cereal-free elimination diet which I have long advised in studying possible food allergy in bronchial asthma and nasal allergy has delayed recognition of foods as a sole cause in 20 to 40 percent of such cases and in varying degrees in association with inhalant allergy in many other patients.*

* *Prevention* Magazine (March 1963).

A lack of the essential fatty acids (vitamin F) and an excess of histamine can be decisive factors in causing asthma. It can come about as a result of chronic infection of the adenoids, sinuses, or tonsils. Some investigators have observed that asthma is worsened by the use of alcoholic beverages and that the inordinate use of salt and sugar aggravates it.

Low blood sugar is a mark of persons with this disease, although it cannot be said to be a cause. It would appear, therefore, that asthmatic attacks are the consequence of more than just one particular deficiency.

While certain drugs, such as cortisone, often give relief, they can also cause considerable harm. Some of the synthetic drugs like aspirin and penicillin may even produce acute asthmatic symptoms in some persons.

Asthma sufferers require many foods high in calcium, iron, and sulphur, in addition to plenty of vitamin C (and I do mean plenty). In attempting to remedy allergies, however, the emphasis should be on a diet fully sufficient in all respects, rather than high in only a few nutrients.

The best protection against allergies is healthy adrenal glands. These glands must be abundantly supplied with vitamin C daily, so that they will continue to produce adrenalin, which detoxifies poisonous material that may have passed into the blood.

Garlic also helps with this trouble, since it has antiseptic properties that suppress disease bacteria in the respiratory tract. Another recommendation is to take a tablespoonful of corn oil at bedtime. Still another encouraging procedure is the use of vitamin E. One hundred units with each meal should be sufficient.

The proper diet gives fine results in most instances, but, to obtain positive and permanent effects, an asthmatic should, first and foremost, make strenuous efforts to abandon the use of all drugs. He should be sure that he is getting a full measure of relaxation, rest, and sleep, to vitalize the nervous system and sustain the general health of the body. Finally, special attention to internal cleansing is imperative for persons who are also susceptible to constipation.

What you eat and drink has a singular influence on your ability to resist respiratory infections, such as bronchitis, colds, hay fever, and influenza. A complete diet high in meat, fish, and eggs is necessary.

Prevention of these illnesses is not too difficult if you eat wisely. However, if you should happen to come down with one of these ailments, you can get excellent results with the following procedure: At the first sign of infection, take substantial doses of a natural vitamin C—say, one thousand milligrams every hour until relief is obtained. By using a natural product, you will also get the bioflavonoids, which are associated with vitamin C and are extremely potent against respiratory diseases. About fifty thousand units of vitamin A should also be taken with each meal.

Another valuable supplement is the enzyme bromelain, found in the pineapple plant. It is marketed through health food and diet shops as a digestive aid, but it has been reported that many people taking bromelain for this purpose have discovered that this oral preparation also has a remarkable effect in the treatment of inflammation resulting from abscesses, arthritis, bronchitis, pneumonia, skin infections, and streptoccal and staph infections, as well as other virulent diseases. According to medical authorities, this catalytic agent reduces inflammation, eases pain, accelerates tissue repair, and substantially shortens recovery time.

Honey, taken frequently during the course of a cold,

is great for breaking up head and chest congestion and expelling phlegm. There's nothing like it. It will help get you better—fast!

Pulmonary emphysema is a condition in which the exceedingly small air sacs in the lungs, from which oxygen is passed on to the blood, break down and become congealed or condensed. Scar tissue builds up, and the patient has difficulty in inhaling and exhaling air completely. Basically, pulmonary emphysema is a persistent inability to expel all the air from the lungs.

More than a million people in the United States are afflicted with this distressing condition, and, in the past ten years, the percentage of deaths it has caused has more than doubled. It is now the chief killer among the lung disorders, causing more deaths than tuberculosis and lung cancer combined. It has also been reported by researchers that chronic emphysema is only exceeded by heart trouble in causing disability in those well along in years.

Shortness of breath is its most conspicuous characteristic, accompanied at times by chronic cough, choking sensation, and heavy breathing. Some cases have responded favorably to exercise and physical therapy.

Concentrated air pollution, such as smog; certain occupational conditions; and cigarette smoking are believed to be active influences in causing this disease.

14

RHEUMATIC INFIRMITIES—NO CAUSE FOR DESPAIR!

WHEN the blood attains a high degree of alkalinity, the accumulation of calcium deposits in the blood-vessel walls is expedited. When this condition reaches its peak, excess calcium or lime begins to settle in the joints, producing arthritis, bursitis, and other rheumatic conditions.

Arthritis is only a new name for what used to be known as rheumatism. It can refer to many different conditions characterized by pain and swelling in the joints of the body.

Sometimes arthritis starts after a heavy cold, tonsilitis, or a gall bladder infection; in many cases, it follows an accidental injury, such as a fracture. Bursitis, gout, muscular rheumatism, osteoarthritis, and rheumatoid arthritis are all manifestations of basically the same disease. Further, osteoarthritis is about twenty times more rampant than the rheumatoid type, which is a wasting disease affecting younger people. The cause is not entirely known. These are ordinarily considered conditions about which little or nothing can be done, and are frequently ailments of long standing.

Although arthritis seems to be largely a disease of elderly people, it is not uncommon for it to afflict persons under forty-five, and even teenage children. One report states that about fifty thousand children in the United States have rheumatoid arthritis. Another recent report from the National Center for Health Statistics declares that over one third of adult Americans suffer to some degree from this disease in one or another of its various manifestations.

It has been noticed in medical circles that arthritics have a proneness to hypoglycemia (low blood sugar). The tremendous increase in arthritic cases in the United States may therefore be partly attributable to the excessive use of refined sugar.

While little is really known about arthritis, it appears that this illness is especially connected with a deficiency of vitamin C. It seems that an insufficiency of this vitamin favors the development of arthritis. If you want to get substantial amounts of vitamin C, eat cabbage, potatoes, red and green peppers, sprouts, tomatoes, and other green vegetables; rose-hip products should also be used. By all means, use optimum quantities of vitamin C daily.

Persons with rheumatic diseases are generally regarded as being calcium-deficient, despite the fact that they are inclined to store up excess calcium. Calcium is one of the best natural pain relievers, so this mineral should not be neglected. Yogurt is a good source. Others are bone meal, blackstrap molasses, and kelp.

Another very valuable addition to the diet of the arthritic is sunflower seeds. In addition to supplying the B vitamins, they are reported to be effective in lessening pain.

In a round of tests on one hundred arthritics, vitamin E therapy was followed by improvement in their symptoms.

Cherries in sizable amounts in the diet have helped

some people—and many have had good results on the simple rule of no sugar.

Many people, especially beekeepers, claim that honey prevents and often cures arthritic and rheumatic ailments. Dr. Melvin Page, D.D.S., author of *Degeneration—Regeneration,* advised his arthritic patients to cut out refined white sugar substances and to take "one tablespoon of molasses or pure honey following each meal. After following the diet for a short time, the patients experienced blessed relief from painful symptoms; most important, their calcium-phosphorus balance was normalized."*

Essential in the treatment of osteoarthritis, rheumatoid arthritis, and other rheumatic conditions is a high-protein diet, because effective nutrition is a must in dealing with any disease. Amino acids are required to build and repair the cells and tissues of the body, particularly around the joints. This means that fresh meat (nothing canned, dried, pickled, or spiced), should predominate in the diet, for the reason that fresh meat is the very best source of these acids. So increase your consumption of meat. As we have noted previously, eggs and fish are also excellent protein foods, and they also supply minerals that are very necessary to combat rheumatic conditions.

Meat (which should not be too well done, so that you will obtain the highest nutritional value) or fish, a freshly baked or boiled potato (unsalted), and a green or yellow vegetable if desired make up a protein dinner of great worth.

If you have arthritis, however, keep citrus fruits and juices out of your diet, as they contain excessive amounts of alkaline minerals, which are apt to produce pain in the joints, aggravating your condition. Likewise, eliminate

* Melvin Page, *Degeneration—Regeneration* (St. Petersburg, Fla.: Biochemical Research Foundation, 1949).

bread and other white flour products. It has been medically recorded that there is a higher incidence of rheumatoid arthritis among people who use wheat foods, which contain gluten, a constituent of wheat flour. Many persons are unable to metabolize gluten, and this leads to chronic inflammation in the intestines, which, it is believed, gradually extends to the joints and lays the foundation for rheumatoid arthritis.

While recovery from chronic arthritis is not usually one of continual forward progress, a fatalistic attitude would be unreasonable. Sometimes a person's body needs to be entirely rebuilt; other cases can be successfully treated by reviving normal circulation around the affected parts. Bear in mind that the faculties of the body are always striving to support and preserve life.

To summarize, then: certain foods are specifically recommended for those suffering from any type of rheumatic condition. The high-protein dietary that follows will maintain the blood sugar at the proper level, which is basic to good health.

BREAKFAST
Four-ounce glass of vegetable juice
Eggs with bacon, ham, or other meat
Coffee or tea (without sugar or cream),
      if desired*

LUNCH
Meat, fish, eggs, or cheese
Lettuce and tomato or a tossed salad
Vegetables
Coffee or tea (without sugar or cream),
      if desired*

* Fruit juices (except citrus fruit juices) may be substituted for coffee or tea at meals, if you wish.

DINNER
Soup (not thickened with flour), if
  desired
Generous portion of meat, fish, or poultry
Vegetables
Coffee or tea (without sugar or cream), if
    desired*

SUITABLE DESSERTS
  Fruit, gelatin, or junket

BETWEEN-MEAL SNACKS
  Fruit juices (except citrus fruit juices), cottage cheese, nuts, seeds, or yogurt are permissible for snacks and before bedtime

SAY "NO" TO
  Bread, cake, and other wheat products, candy, soft drinks, ice cream, macaroni, spaghetti, pastries, pies, puddings, and refined white sugar

Add the following nutrients to your diet, and you will be bound to get a favorable response:

APPLE CIDER VINEGAR WITH HONEY
  Minerals are essential for the relief of rheumatic conditions. A tablespoonful of apple cider vinegar combined with a tablespoonful of honey in a glass of water twice a day will supply minerals, vitamins, and enzymes. When this remedy is taken, any excess calcium in the joints enters into solution with the blood.

BONE MEAL
  It is a high-quality source of calcium and phosphorus, as well as all the trace minerals.

BREWER'S YEAST
  One of the best sources of protein, including the amino acids (necessary in the treatment of arthritis), and minerals, it can be added to other foods to boost their protein content.

  * Fruit juices (except citrus fruit juices) may be substituted for coffee or tea at meals, if you wish.

KELP

Sea kelp contains a naturally balanced combination of sixty minerals, twelve vitamins, and twenty-one amino acids.

SUNFLOWER SEEDS

One of the most perfect foods known, they are reported to diminish the pain of arthritis.

VITAMIN A

This vitamin is extremely valuable for the health of all the body organs and particularly as a deterrent of infections.

VITAMIN C

Vitamin C is absolutely necessary for the durability of blood-vessel walls and is required to bind the cells in the tissues together. It is effective in treating arthritis.

VITAMIN P (THE BIOFLAVONOIDS)

This vitamin is part of the vitamin C complex. Be sure to use a vitamin C product that includes the bioflavonoids.

15

UNDERSTANDING SUCCESSFUL WEIGHT REDUCTION

IS overweight hereditary? Perhaps, but only to the degree that body build is inherited. Weight control, like other good health practices, begins with knowledge of proper nutrition. Merely counting calories is not the most practical way to slenderize. Eating the right foods will stimulate the thyroid gland to secrete more of the hormone that maintains normal weight, and this will automatically tend to regulate your weight.

Obesity is as notable a symptom of a lack of proper nutrition as is underweight, and almost everyone will agree that this condition shortens life. Overweight is a widespread disorder in civilized nations, but it does not prevail among primitive races living on simple diets.

Needless to say, obesity is injurious to health in many ways. It increases the risk of damage to the arteries, the kidneys, and especially the heart. It is now known to have a bearing on the cancer death rate as well. Surveys conducted by life insurance companies indicate that overweight people of advanced age are more likely to die of cancer than those of average weight. The United States

149

Department of Agriculture has called overweight "probably the chief dietary hazard of modern living."

As to the cause of overweight, Adelle Davis, a leading nutritionist, writes:

> There are many causes. One, I suspect, is that our foods are so depleted of the nutrients which starved bodies crave that overeating is due to a physiological compulsion to obtain them; even that usually fails to supply the nutrients longed for by the tissues. Another cause is that people often eat too little rather than too much; the basal metabolism drops far below normal; there is no energy for work or play, none to be turned into heat. When few calories are used, few are needed.[1]

The rate of metabolism has a bearing on whether a person is fat or slender, and this is controlled essentially by the kind of food one consumes. Certain nutrients are necessary for speedy metabolism, principally calcium, iodine, and iron. The thyroid gland, which controls the speed of metabolic processes, needs, in addition to iodine, zinc and certain B vitamins.

Some persons are overweight due to the retention of excess water in the tissues, because their protein consumption is insufficient. They generally have inferior health and a greater susceptibility to degenerative diseases. When the proper foods are supplied, however, the body sheds this fat and water.

If you are troubled with overweight, hold to a high-protein diet and take moderate exercise. If you also make sure to use the foods that offer the best sources of minerals and vitamins, the chances are good that your excess weight will come off and stay off. Furthermore, you will be obtaining the carbohydrates in the variety and form in which you are intended to get them. Since these will be

[1] Adelle Davis, *Let's Eat Right to Keep Fit* (New York: Harcourt, Brace & World, 1954).

the right sort of starches and sugars, you will not have to be too concerned about calories. Good food is fuel for the body. There is no need to go off the deep end by starving off extra weight.

Older people should bear in mind that, because their metabolic activity, as well as all the other physical functions, is slowed down, trying to lose excess weight will be more difficult for them.

The foremost enemies of proper weight are white flour products, fried foods, salt, and sugar. If you wish to reduce, you must give up foods like bread, cake, candy, cookies, ice cream, pastries, and rich dressings and sauces. It is not generally known, for example, that a stick of chewing gum contains 63 percent sugar and 16 percent corn syrup. One stick is enough to halt weight loss. Such "foods" are practically dead as far as vitamins and minerals are concerned. Substitute complete protein foods, such as eggs, fish, and meat, together with cottage cheese, fresh fruits, green vegetables, and yogurt.

During the past several years, my experience has been that adherence to a high-protein, high-fat diet, enriched with the necessary nutrients, is the most feasible method of preventing a weight problem. I have actually lost weight, and my waist measurement has dropped two inches, since I began following this diet.

An all-meat diet is wholesome and takes very little time to prepare. Restricting vegetables and salads, and cutting out elaborate desserts, lowers the cost per meal to a moderate sum.

Wine, in addition to aiding in digestion of foods, has been found effective in causing weight reduction.

It has been reported in the *New York State Journal of Medicine*, November 1, 1962, that discreet use of wine with dinner has resulted in a more rapid loss of body weight in obese people, and particularly in those who are a victim of compulsive raiding of the refrigerator at night. Subjects given wine with dinner or before bedtime lost almost twice as much weight per week as subjects who were given the same meals without the wine. . . . Those troubled with compulsive eating were given more will-power by the wine, and were benefited in alleviation of insomnia.[2]

For many years, Dr. Blake F. Donaldson, a distinguished New York physician, has efficiently treated overweight people with a dietary in which up to twenty-four ounces of fat meat were permitted daily.

First, he prescribes a thirty-minute walk before breakfast. This, he says, is extremely important. Second, he recommends an exclusive diet of one half-pound of fat meat (any kind), with a half-cup of black coffee, if desired, three times a day. To this is added three glasses of water between meals, three in the morning, and three in the afternoon. No water is allowed after five o'clock. As the patient improves, the doctor allows the addition of a baked potato, fruit, and sometimes an additional vegetable. Finally, he prohibits sugar, seltzer and carbonated drinks, bread (any kind), flour products, and alcohol.[3]

If you have vainly tried to reduce your weight, be assured that you can lower it. A reduction in weight will greatly improve your health and will ease the strain on your heart. This becomes a goal well worth working for when one realizes that deaths from hardening of the arteries, high blood pressure, and heart disease are two and a half times as great among overweight people as they are among those of normal weight.

In truth, the only solution to the problem is to make a practice of eating only natural foods, high in vitamins and

[2] *Health and Nutrition News* (May 1963).
[3] Blake F. Donaldson, *Strong Medicine* (Garden City, N.Y.: Doubleday & Co., 1962).

minerals, so that the smallest quantity of food will suffice. There is no other way. If you wish to lose weight, here are three points to remember:

EAT PROTEIN FOODS.

STOP EATING FANCY DESSERTS.

DRINK COFFEE WITHOUT CREAM AND SUGAR.

Try it. It works—naturally!

16

FINISH STRONGER, LIVE LONGER

IN the preceding pages, I have mainly been concerned with the needs of the body, how it should be nurtured and cared for so as to keep it strong and free from disease. Whether or not you have a health problem, I can assure you that you will never regret adopting at least the salient features of the food regimen I have proposed. If you do, you will find, as I did, that your initiative and willingness to make a venture have been well rewarded.

Current studies of longevity provide no ground for the belief that sudden breakdowns in health must be expected at any certain age. A human being matures in about twenty-five years and, with reasonable care, should live to be one hundred years old or even older. Our bodies can retain their vitality even into the second century, without wearing out in any essential part.

Reasonable living and good nutrition are of major importance for health and appearance, and, if practiced diligently, they will pay off in dramatically improved well-being. Bear in mind that one cannot disregard the laws of health and then repair the error by taking a couple of pills.

Look for the flaws in your daily meals, then take the simple steps I have outlined for building health and resistance to disease. You must act now to accomplish changes for the better. You should aim for all-round good nutrition, remembering that no one vitamin or mineral can do everything.

If you are still young—that is, between forty and sixty—you should know that your health is in your own hands. You can prolong the middle years, which can be the best years of your life. This is not a vague promise. The connection between food and health is proven, and it merits your serious consideration. Aristotle said that if there is one way that is better than another, it is the way of nature.

If you will put your knowledge of nutrition to work during these intermediate years, you will greatly improve your chances of having a long and healthy old age. Don't forget that, no matter what your age, the body never loses its inherent ability to recuperate—if you give it a chance.

Good health, however, may be practically impossible to attain unless one combines with it an equally sound mind. There is an interdependence of the physical and the spiritual, and health means the precise harmony of both. Not everything in life is under the control of material forces that cannot be resisted. Much worry and anxiety is born of fatigue, and this is generally acknowledged to be the most baneful influence that threatens the mind of man. Recent research into chemical influences on the brain indicates that many unwholesome and disruptive emotions arise out of alterations in body chemistry due to faulty eating habits, low blood sugar, and inadequate sleep. Such physical and psychological ills include anxiety, depression, discouragement, high blood pressure, self-pity, ulcers, and unhappiness: indeed, all of these, which testify to the inevitable power of the mind over the body, embitter and impair the integrity of the human organism. Make sure, then, that you are healthy in body and in soul.

Be confident, therefore—and take heart. At long last, you have found the key to a new power and a new life—not in some shadowy, uncertain tomorrow, but today. Now!

SUGGESTED READING

THIS bibliography is not intended to be all-inclusive. Each book or magazine that you read will lead you to others.

BOOKS

Abrahamson, E. M., and A. W. Pezet. *Body, Mind and Sugar.* New York: Holt, Rinehart & Winston, 1951.

Bailey, Herbert. *Vitamin E: Your Key to a Healthy Heart.* New York: Arc Books, 1967.

Beck, Bodog F., and Doree Smedley. *Honey and Your Health.* New York: Dodd, Mead, 1944.

Blaine, Tom R. *Goodbye Allergies.* New York: The Citadel Press, 1965.

Clark, Linda. *Stay Young Longer.* New York: The Devin-Adair Co., 1962.

Cummings, Robert. *Stay Young and Vital.* Englewood Cliffs, N.J.: Prentice-Hall, 1960.

Davis, Adelle. *Let's Eat Right to Keep Fit.* New York: Harcourt, Brace & World, 1954.

———. *You Can Stay Well.* Chicago, Ill.: Frederick H. Bartz, 1959.

Donaldson, Blake F. *Strong Medicine.* Garden City, New York: Doubleday & Co., 1962.

Elwood, Cathryn. *Feel Like a Million.* New York: The Devin-Adair Co., 1958.

Fredericks, Carlton. *Eat, Live and Be Merry.* New York: Paxton-Slade Publishing Co., 1961.

Fredericks, Carlton, and Herbert Bailey. *Food Facts and Fallacies.* New York: Arc Books, 1968.

Hunter, Kathleen. *Health Foods and Herbs.* New York: Arc Books, 1963.

Hauser, Gayelord. *Look Younger, Live Longer.* New York: Farrar, Straus, & Co., 1951.

Jarvis, D. C. *Arthritis and Folk Medicine.* New York: Holt, Rinehart & Winston, 1960.

————. *Folk Medicine.* New York: Holt, Rinehart & Winston, 1958.

Loughran, John X. *Formula for Genius.* New York: The Devin-Adair Co., 1964.

————. *90 Days to a Better Heart.* New York: The Devin-Adair Co., 1958.

Mackarness, Richard. *Eat Fat and Grow Slim.* Garden City, N.Y.: Doubleday & Co., 1959.

Rodale, J. I. *The Prevention Method for Better Health.* Emmaus, Penna.: Rodale Books, 1960.

————. *Skits and Conversations Towards Better Healh.* Emmaus, Penna.: Rodale Books, 1958.

Shute, Drs. Evan and Wilfred. *Your Heart and Vitamin E.* Detroit, Mich.: The Cardiac Society, 1956.

Townsend, Richard D. *Let's Talk Health Sense.* Boston, Mass.: Bruce-Humphries, 1960.

MAGAZINES

Health Bulletin (Robert Rodale, ed., Rodale Press, Inc., Emmaus, Penna.).

Health and Nutrition News (Carlton Fredericks, ed., Box 10, Midtown Station, New York, N. Y.).

Health Saver Magazine (Roland E. Horvath, ed. dir., Hackensack, N.J.).

Prevention Magazine (J. I. Rodale, ed., Emmaus, Penna.).

Note: Practically all the titles listed are available at health food and diet shops everywhere.